BILL OF RIGHT KNOW THYSELF

BLACK WHITE & SHADOWS OF HUMANITY
HEALTH HERITAGE

NEUROSCIENCE

PHILOSOPHY

HUMANITY

ENGLISH VERSION

AUTHOR BY:

Lorenzi R. Marcos

Get in touch with Authors through this Provided Email/Website and social media handle and learn more about the inner discovery and health fitness :

http://healthwisetrainer.com

Lorenzipersonaltrainer@gmail.com

IG: lorenzi_marcos

info@healthwisetrainer.com

Lorenzi R.Marcos

WHO WHEN

BILL OF RIGHTS

You

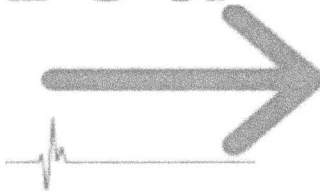

Them

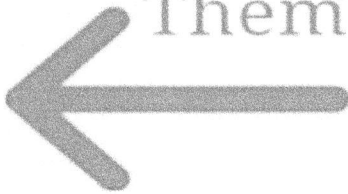

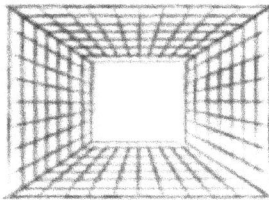

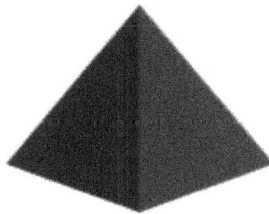

LORENZI R. MARCOS

Contents

DISCLAIMER

This publication offers science-based insights to enhance overall health and promote healthy lifestyle choices for adults aged 18-65. It does not seek to supplant professional medical advice or treatment. The author advises readers to consult qualified healthcare professionals for personalized guidance concerning specific health concerns.

Key Points:

- **Scientific Foundation:** All information is grounded in credible scientific research and evidence.

- **Target Audience:** This eBook is for adults aged 18 to 65 who seek to enhance their overall health and well-being.

- **Not a Substitute for Medical Advice:** Readers are urged to seek expert medical advice before making significant lifestyle changes or addressing specific health concerns.

- **Holistic Approach:** The book addresses three fundamental aspects of holistic health: mindset (incorporating neuroscience and mindfulness philosophy), nutrition (emphasizing healthy choices and sustainability), and fitness (understanding various muscle groups and their functions).

- **Individual Consideration:** While readers of all abilities, limitations, medical conditions, or ages beyond the target range are welcome to glean insights from this book, unique circumstances may necessitate additional or specialized guidance.

Exploring Options and Embracing Support:

This book introduces readers to scientifically backed strategies and approaches tailored to their current transition phase. It highlights:

- The role of qualified therapists and counselors is to offer personalized guidance and support, including cognitive behavioral therapy (CBT) and other evidence-based interventions.

- The potential benefits of connecting with others facing similar challenges for understanding, encouragement, and mutual accountability.

- The importance of incorporating nourishing activities, cultivating positive relationships, and addressing underlying mental health concerns to fortify the foundation for well-being.

A Detailed Path to Transformation:

Taking a comprehensive approach, the book underscores how:

- Skill-building fosters a growth-oriented mindset, enabling resilience in the face of setbacks and reframing challenges as opportunities for growth.

- Nourishing the body with wholesome foods sustains energy levels and mood, laying the groundwork for lasting change.

- Regular physical activity enhances self-efficacy, stress management, and overall well-being, generating positive effects across various aspects of life.

This book integrates these elements within the Transtheoretical Model (TTM) framework to offer a comprehensive roadmap for long-term transformation. Whether contemplating change or actively planning your journey, it is your companion, guide, and supporter in unlocking your full potential.

Breaking Free from Negative Habits and Addiction:

Breaking free from negative habits and addiction is a complex process, often marked by internal resistance and external pressures.

The Transtheoretical Model (TTM), pioneered by James Prochaska and Carlo DiClemente, provides a valuable framework for understanding and facilitating individual behavior modification. Its dynamic and unbiased approach acknowledges the non-linear nature of change, recognizing that individuals progress through different stages at their own pace.

CHAPTER 1

INTRODUCTION

Welcome, fellow traveler, to a notable adventure through the realms of notions meticulously crafted by Marcos R. Lorenzi. Prepare to embark on a highbrow odyssey wherein entrenched biases are confronted, minds are liberated from conformity, and a transformative quest for knowledge unfolds.

This narrative is neither predetermined nor seeks to impose an unmarried, prevalent solution. Within these pages lies a vibrant tapestry woven from numerous perspectives, each meticulously tested and presented with profound recognition. Like a pro cartographer, the author navigates the considerable panorama of human experience, exploring the intricacies of nutrition, the workings of the mind, and the captivating narratives of records and society.

Crucially, this day trip goes beyond self-diagnosis and brief fixes. It empowers you, the discerning reader, to method every idea significantly, fostering a deep understanding of our complex global realities. This transformative voyage encourages you to embrace specialists' knowledge while remaining vigilant toward societal manipulation.

As you embark on this intellectual journey, remember that the understanding won is not passive but a catalyst for self-discovery and acceptable change. Allow yourself to be captivated by various perspectives, challenge established beliefs with intellectual rigor, and emerge with an empowered sense of curiosity and a renewed appreciation for the potential of the human spirit.

Bon voyage!

REINTRODUCTION OF THE "PUZZLE" METAPHOR

Join me on this expedition, not as a patient seeking treatment but as a fellow voyager on self-discovery! Let's unearth the hero within, one puzzle piece at a time!

Envision your life as a magnificent mosaic, yet some pieces still need to be added or marred! This guide will aid you in locating those missing fragments — mindset, mindfulness, nutrition, fitness, philosophy, and history — and demonstrate how to fit them together to realize your ideal self.

Cast aside overwhelming theories and convoluted jargon! This journey entails taking small, deliberate steps leading to enduring change. In every chapter, you'll encounter simple exercises, actionable tips, and pragmatic tools designed to help you integrate these fundamental elements into your daily routine. It's not merely about inundating yourself with information; it's about introspection and transformation. You'll find opportunities to journal, meditate, and explore your experiences through thought-provoking prompts and questions.

Throughout our expedition, you'll possess a robust "Toolbox" with holistic, evidence-based strategies for sustainable health and well-being. These options provide a secure pathway for crafting your unique journey to success.

CHAPTER 2

UNDERSTANDING THE STAGES OF CHANGE THE EMPOWERING POTENTIAL OF THE TTM

The Transtheoretical Model (TTM) identifies six stages of change: pre-contemplation, contemplation, preparation, action, maintenance, and termination. Focusing on the initial three stages in this book allows for a tailored approach suited to individuals at the outset of their transformation journey.

Exploring Processes of Change: Additionally, the TTM identifies ten "processes of change" — specific strategies individuals employ to navigate each stage. By addressing these processes in your book, readers can acquire tools to confront challenges and progress forward. For instance, during the preparation stage, individuals might utilize consciousness-raising to gather information about healthier alternatives or employ counterconditioning to substitute negative habits with positive ones.

Integration with Mindset, Mindfulness, Nutrition, and Fitness: The TTM's adaptability permits integration with various domains that facilitate positive change. Your book can delve into how fostering a positive mindset aids individuals in embracing setbacks, how practicing mindfulness enhances self-awareness and emotional regulation, how dietary choices impact energy levels and mood, and how engaging in physical activity boosts self-confidence and stress management.

International Resources on the TTM:

- The Pro-Change Behavior Solutions website: Pro-Change Behavior Solutions

- The James Prochaska and Carlo DiClemente Centre for Health Behavior Change: "The Transtheoretical Model of Health Behavior Change" - James O. Prochaska, Wayne F. Velicer, 1997, Sage Publications.

With an understanding of the TTM and a holistic perspective, you'll explore using this framework to unleash your potential for positive change.

APPROACHESS SEARCH FOR THE HERO: AN ANTHEM OF INNER STRENGTH

The inspiring melody "Search for the Hero" was penned by the British dance music band, with Mike Pickering and Paul Heard credited as its composers. Released as a single in 1995, its message of resilience and personal growth transcends time.

Discovering the Hero Within:

At its essence, the song urges listeners to unearth the hero within themselves, the wellspring of strength and potential often obscured by doubt or despair. It acknowledges life's trials, likening them to a "river that flows but nothing breathes" or a "train arriving but never leaving." Despite these challenges, it implores us to maintain faith and "keep on aiming high," viewing self-discovery as the key to unlocking our true essence.

Empowering Lyrics:

Lines such as "Search for the secrets you hide / Search for the hero inside yourself" serve as potent mantras, reminding us that the answers we seek lie within. The song underscores the importance of personal agency, urging us to "seek yourself and you will shine," instilling a sense of empowerment and self-belief.

More Than a Song:

"Search for the Hero" transcends being a pop anthem; it becomes a motivational call to action, reminding us that we possess the inherent ability to overcome adversity. Its message resonates with anyone striving to break free from limitations and unlock their full potential, rendering it a timeless anthem for personal growth and inner strength.

Have you ever been captivated by a song not solely for its melody but for its underlying message? A message that resonates deeply within you, even if you don't fully comprehend the lyrics? That's precisely what happened to me 25 years ago before I even grasped the nuances of English. This song, born from a childhood in Brazil and nurtured in the vibrant streets of Italy, planted the silent seed of a lifelong quest.

Years later, as a personal trainer and weight management specialist, I witnessed countless individuals embark on transformative journeys. Each tale, unique yet familiar, echoed the themes of that age-old song. It was the struggle for change, the battle against ingrained habits and addictions, the yearning to break free and become the best version of oneself.

With the foundation laid and inner strength embraced it's time to ignite the spark within!

This book doesn't promise a quick fix, a miracle cure, or a one-size-fits-all solution. Instead, it invites readers to embark on a voyage of self-discovery, armed with the six pillars of human potential: mindset, mindfulness, nutrition, fitness, neuroscience, and philosophy.

Envision these elements as a complex puzzle, each essential for constructing unwavering well-being.

We'll delve into the science behind mindset shifts, the potency of mindfulness in navigating emotions, the nourishment that fuels both body and mind and the physical prowess that unlocks our potential.

With its timeless wisdom from Stoicism, Buddhism, and Hermeticism, philosophy will guide self-awareness and moderation. At the same time, history, with its tapestry of triumphs and tragedies, reminds us that we are not alone in this quest.

Yet, the true hero of this journey resides within you. This book acts as your map, your compass, but your unwavering spirit will propel you forward. Together, we'll explore the pivotal stages of change, from the initial spark of awareness to the challenges of neuroplasticity, the brain's extraordinary capacity to rewire itself.

We'll acknowledge the societal influences and experiences shaping our present and empower you to delve into their root causes. Comprehending the intricate interplay of environment, genetics, beliefs, nutrition, and even trauma can unlock the potential for positive change.

The world grapples with addiction in its myriad forms – from substances to power, validation, and instant gratification. This book doesn't shy away from these harsh realities; instead, it serves as a beacon of hope, reminding us that our struggles do not define us.

CHAPTER 3

EXPLORING THE TOOLBOX OF SELF FROM TURBULENCE TO TRANQUILITY

For two decades, we've witnessed a cascade of environmental, social, and existential crises sweep across the globe, leaving a trail of devastation in their wake. We're assured that time will heal these wounds, yet for many, the balm of time arrives too late.

Amidst the clamor for a sustainable planet and enduring rights, we posit a new imperative: sustainable embodiment. Only by establishing a resilient mind can we construct a future of flourishing.

Guided by a profound reverence for humanity's well-being and its legacy of healing, unburdened by reactionary impulses, I present The Toolbox Laboratory. The name resonates with the meticulous checks and mindful control of my aviation training, which prevent catastrophic errors.

Each element serves as an instrument for navigating the turbulence within, assembled for your self-discovery.

This isn't merely about survival but soaring above the storms. It's about crafting inner resilience, forging clarity from chaos, and reclaiming the power to heal ourselves and the world.

The Toolbox Laboratory, the dear explorer, awaits your journey to wholeness.

Toolbox N1 for Active Engagement:

1. **Pen and Paper:** Take notes, journal your thoughts, and sketch out personal connections as you progress!

2. **Relaxation Techniques:** Master the 3x6x9 breathing method or explore other mindfulness practices to enhance focus and reduce stress!

Safety Considerations:

- Pre-existing Conditions: Consult a healthcare professional if you have respiratory conditions like asthma, COPD, or high blood pressure!

Lorenzi R.Marcos

- Listen to Your Body: Start with shorter durations and increase gradually. Stop if you feel dizzy or discomfort!

- Focus on Controlled Breathing: Avoid forceful inhalations or exhalations, and ensure your breaths are diaphragmatic (belly breaths)!

Holistic Benefits:
- Reduced Stress and Anxiety: Deep, controlled breathing activates the parasympathetic nervous system, promoting relaxation and lowering stress hormones.

- Improved Focus and Clarity: Focused breathing can clear your mind, enhance concentration, and boost alertness.

- Increased Relaxation and Sleep Quality: Deeper breaths relax the body and mind, leading to better sleep.

Anatomic Viewpoint:
- Diaphragmatic Breathing: Engages the diaphragm muscle, promoting deeper breaths and maximizing oxygen intake.

- Improved Gas Exchange: Better oxygen and carbon dioxide exchange benefits circulation.

- Reduced Tension: Helps release tension in the chest and abdomen, promoting relaxation.

- Additional Notes: Experiment with breath durations to find what's comfortable and practical! Combining this technique with meditation can enhance its benefits.

3. **Posture Awareness:** Check and adjust your posture for optimal comfort and focus! Taking breaks and rejuvenating yourself fuels your learning journey.

4. **Personalized Exploration:** Don't feel overwhelmed by absorbing everything! Identify the elements that resonate most and dive deeper into those areas! Your journey is unique, and each chapter introduces various ideas and resources, empowering you to choose what suits you best.

OBSERVATION, NOT ABSORPTION

Empathy, knowledge, and support are pivotal tools for our exploration in the following sections.

In the flickering fluorescent light of the diner, Liam stirred his coffee, steam swirling like the thoughts in his head. He watched a couple laughing across the booth, their joy contrasting with the knot of tension in his stomach. He yearned for that ease, that lightness, but felt trapped by the invisible chains of his addiction.

Liam's struggle wasn't with food or alcohol but with the siren song of the digital world. Hours have bled into each other, lost in the dopamine rush of likes and notifications. The escape it offered was tempting, masking the anxieties and insecurities that gnawed at him. Yet, the emptiness that followed each digital binge left him feeling unmoored, further from the life he desired.

Across town, Sarah sat in her dimly lit apartment, the silence broken only by the click of her keyboard. Each line of code she wrote fed a different hunger – the need for validation, the fear of failure, the constant pressure to achieve. Food had become her silent companion, a source of comfort and a burden on her body and spirit. The cycle of guilt and shame felt endless, a hamster wheel of self-destruction.

Miles away, Ben gripped the steering wheel, knuckles white. The world sped by in a blur as he pushed the accelerator further, chasing the thrill of speed. It was a fleeting escape from the pressures of work, the doubts about his relationship, and the constant feeling of being on the edge. But the adrenaline high always gave way to a bone-deep fear, a stark reminder of the risks he was taking.

These were just three stories woven from different threads of struggle with online addiction, emotional eating, and compulsive behaviors. Yet, they shared a common thread: the yearning for change, the fight against the forces that held them captive.

Their journeys wouldn't be easy. There would be stumbles, moments of doubt, and the ever-present pull of their addictions.

Lorenzi R.Marcos

But within each of them flickered a spark of hope fueled by the knowledge that they weren't alone.

Liam sought the support of a therapy group, finding strength in shared experiences and the wisdom of others. Sarah explored mindfulness practices, learning to soothe her anxieties without turning to food. Ben joined a running club, channeling his need for speed into a healthier pursuit. Their paths were diverse, but the tools they used were universal. Mindfulness helped them recognize triggers and choose different responses. Self-awareness allowed them to understand the root causes of their addictions. Discipline became their ally, guiding them towards healthier choices.

They discovered their brains' neuroplasticity, learning that change was possible, one step at a time. They drew strength from philosophy, finding solace in Stoic principles of acceptance and Buddhist teachings on compassion. History offered them perspective, reminding them that countless others had walked this path before.

Their transformations weren't linear but a tapestry woven with setbacks and triumphs. They learned to celebrate minor victories, like waking up before dawn for a run, attending a therapy session, or resisting the urge to scroll.

While they had distinct stories, they resonated with others facing similar battles. Their different stories demonstrated that freedom was possible, becoming beacons of hope and proof that even the most ingrained patterns could be broken. Their journeys weren't over, but they had taken the first step, the most important one—the step toward themselves.

CHAPTER 4

INDIVIDUAL CASE STUDIES AND THE IMPLICATIONS OF NEUROPLASTICITY

This chapter presents three individual case studies of individuals who successfully overcame addiction through various methods. These accounts are provided solely for illustrative purposes and are not intended to serve as medical, psychological, or spiritual advice.

It is essential to recognize that the experiences and solutions depicted in these case studies are unique and may not resonate with every reader's journey. While the book explores neuroplasticity, which refers to the brain's ability to rewire, it is crucial to understand that individual outcomes will vary based on several factors. These include the severity and nature of the addiction, the individual's existing mental and physical health conditions, and the specific approaches and support systems utilized.

Furthermore, this book references aspects of Stoicism, Buddhism, and scientific research in their potential relevance to navigating challenging personal journeys. However, these references are intended solely to stimulate discussion and broaden perspectives. The book does not advocate or endorse any particular belief system or therapy as a universal solution for addiction.

The author emphasizes that mentioning these philosophical schools and research is not meant to establish any causal or prescriptive relationship between them and the case studies presented.

Ultimately, the book aims to facilitate individual exploration and encourage readers to seek professional guidance tailored to their needs. It is strongly advised to consult qualified healthcare professionals before changing health and wellness routines.

CHAPTER 5

BREAK FREE FROM THE ILLUSION: RECLAIM YOUR JOURNEY WITH SUSTAINABLE CHANGE

Are you tired of chasing after quick fixes and false promises in your battle against addiction? This book offers something different. It's about empowering you to carve out your unique path to well-being, customized to address your needs and challenges.

We understand the real struggles. Addiction affects individuals from all walks of life, and access to healthcare and resources can vary widely, adding further obstacles to the journey of recovery. This book acknowledges these disparities and aims to provide a universally accessible roadmap, irrespective of background or circumstances.

Here's what sets this book apart:

- **Holistic and Safe Approach:** We move away from the one-size-fits-all approach and focus on sustainable, holistic practices that nurture your mind, body, and spirit. By integrating mindfulness, nutrition, movement, and self-compassion, you lay the groundwork for lasting change.

- **Professional Guidance, Always:** This book underscores the critical role of qualified professionals in supporting your journey. While offering practical tools and insights, it stresses the importance of seeking expert guidance, especially for specific health conditions.

- **Respecting Your Pace:** Transformation is a gradual process. This book encourages you to honor your body's natural rhythms and resist the allure of quick fixes. Sustainable change requires patience and perseverance, and we celebrate every step of your journey.

- **Empowering, Not Exploiting:** Say goodbye to self-proclaimed gurus and gimmicks! This book is about dispelling the clouds of misinformation and empowering you to reclaim control over your well-being. It's about recognizing your inner strength and harnessing it for positive change. You can transform your life regardless of your financial limitations, beliefs, or location. This book serves as a supportive companion, guiding you through the complexities of addiction recovery with a holistic, mindful approach. Whether embarking on your journey or seeking a renewed sense of motivation, these pages offer a haven for self-discovery and sustainable growth.

RISE, BREAK FREE: UNLEASH YOUR POTENTIAL BEYOND THE NOISE!

Let's draw inspiration from Nikola Tesla's wisdom, "If you want to find the secrets of the universe, think in terms of energy, frequency, and vibration." Consider the demonstrated connection between thought and ATP consumption in the brain! Could directing our thoughts and intentions toward specific frequencies or vibrations potentially influence our cognitive abilities, emotions, or overall well-being? If so, how might we explore this concept through scientific inquiry or personal experimentation?

REFLECTION ON THE QUOTE

Tesla's provocative statement invites us to shift our perspective beyond the tangible and delve into the unseen forces that shape our reality. While scientific understanding of energy, frequency, and vibration primarily focuses on physical phenomena, could their influence extend to consciousness and thought? Our thoughts and emotions, like tiny oscillators, resonate at different frequencies, impacting how we interact with the world and ourselves. If so, could consciously tuning these frequencies offer a pathway to self-improvement, healing, or unlocking hidden potential?

STUDIES

- Raichle, M. E. (1994). Images of brain function. Proceedings of the National Academy of Sciences, 91(25), 12009-12014. Link

- Logothetis, N. K. et al. (2001). Neurobiological basis of the brain's capacity for complex visual processing. Nature, 412(6845), 545-549. Link

Note: It's important to remember that Tesla's quote and the concept of "frequency" in the context of consciousness are not directly supported by mainstream science. However, they can serve as starting points for open-ended exploration and discussion.

Matthew 22:37-39: "Jesus replied: 'Love the Lord your God with all your heart and with all your soul and with all your mind.' '"

CHAPTER 6

THE POWER OF 12 DAYS: A CATALYST FOR EXPLORATION

Building upon the foundation of the previous chapters, we embark on a 12-day journey of self-discovery, using open-ended questions to spark introspection and curiosity.

1. **Navigating Crossroads:** What internal compass guides your decisions as you stand at this junction in your life? What values or desires whisper the direction you truly want to go?

2. **Rewiring Synapses:** Your brain constantly rewires itself based on experiences. What intentional thoughts, actions, or habits could you nurture to cultivate your desired neural pathways?

3. **Observing the Observer:** When faced with challenges, do you become consumed by the storm or step back to observe your reactions with detached curiosity? Can you cultivate the ability to witness your thoughts and emotions without judgment?

4. **The Power of Perception:** How do you frame your current situation? Can reframing your internal narrative, focusing on opportunities for growth rather than limitations, empower you?

5. **Seeking Sanctuary:** Where do you find inner peace and clarity moments? Can nurturing these sanctuaries, be it mindfulness practice, connecting with nature, or creative expression, offer refuge and renewal?

6. **Kindness Towards Self:** We all stumble. How can you cultivate self-compassion, treating yourself with the same gentle understanding you would offer a cherished friend facing similar struggles?

7. **Fueling Potential:** What ignites your curiosity and sparks joy? Exploring activities that tap into your intrinsic motivation can nourish your spirit and fuel your journey.

8. **Gratitude's Garden:** Reflecting on what you appreciate, even amidst challenges, can cultivate a more positive outlook. What small blessings might you overlook in your daily routine?

9. **Learning from Experience:** Every challenge holds lessons. Can you identify the wisdom gleaned from past struggles that can guide you forward with greater resilience?

10. **Building Your Support Network:** Who uplifts and inspires you? Can fostering more profound connections with these individuals or seeking supportive communities provide strength and encouragement?

11. **Celebrating Small Victories:** Progress often unfolds in subtle ways. Can you acknowledge and celebrate your small triumphs to fuel your motivation, no matter how seemingly insignificant?

12. **Embracing the Unknown:** The future is uncharted. How can you cultivate a sense of adventure and openness to learning and growth as you navigate the uncertainties?

(You might think this is about another super method crafted by a guru with its extraordinary discovery; however, it is far from this scenario; my stoic principles were not found on a BLACK FRIDAY, so be patient to craft your perception.)

CHAPTER 7

BREAKING FREE: EMBRACING YOUR JOURNEY TO SELF-DISCOVERY

Imagine a canvas smudged with the hues of addiction and negativity! Within this canvas lies a weary but undefeated hero yearning to break free. This is your story, a tale whispered by your soul. But fear not! For the path to liberation isn't paved with suffering. It's a dance of self-love and divine consciousness, an expedition where time becomes your ally, not your enemy. Forget the promises of cures and miracle fixes! This journey demands no sacrifice, no penance, just a gentle invitation to turn inwards. It's a holiday from the past, a bridge to the future, built with the bricks of present awareness. Here, you'll shed the weight of worry, guilt, and shame, leaving only the lightness of self-discovery. Think of these days as a gift, a chance to unwrap your true essence! Put down the books, the certifications, and the labels! This is a journey of the soul, guided by the whispers of your divine spark. Each day, your journal becomes your confidant, a canvas where you paint the colors of your awakening.

> **Embrace the Symphony of Senses!** Your mind will no longer be a fog-shrouded landscape. Throw open the windows and let the fresh air of awareness cleanse your thoughts! Savor the new flavors of your emotions and breathe in the fragrance of possibilities! Each sense becomes a portal to your inner world, revealing hidden strengths and forgotten passions.

> **Silence the Chorus of Doubt!** Fear and anxiety cling to you like shadows, whispering tales of failure. But remember! The hero within is not defined by their battles but by their resilience. In this haven of self-love, there's no room for judgment, only space for acceptance and growth.

> **Friendly with the Unknown!** The path may not be linear, and the destination may be uncertain. But isn't that the beauty of life? Embrace the unknown! Let curiosity be your

compass! Each step and discovery uncover a more profound truth about yourself, leading you closer to the light of freedom. Remember, dear reader! You are not alone. This is a collective dance, a chorus of souls seeking liberation. Join the movement, share your story, and let your light inspire others! This 12-day journey is not just a program; it's a revolution within. It's a call to silence the external noise and awaken the hero within. So, take a breath, step onto the canvas, and paint your masterpiece of self-discovery! The time for change is now, and the brush is in your hand.

"Virtue alone is happiness, and wickedness alone is misery."
Hierocles, Discourses (2nd century AD)

Let's explore our best friends in the following chapters with silence, conscious breathing, an open mind, and a sage half glass with pure Crystal water where only the necessary will be added!

CHAPTER 8

AN OVERVIEW OF PHILOSOPHY

Philosophy, deriving from the Greek "Philia" (love) and "Sophia" (wisdom), is a multifaceted pursuit unlike any other. It does not seek definitive answers like science nor preach dogma like religion. Instead, it continually examines existence, knowledge, and the human condition driven by curiosity and reason.

The seeds of philosophy were planted in ancient Greece, where luminaries like Socrates, Plato, and Aristotle pondered fundamental questions about reality, ethics, and justice. Socrates focused on questioning and self-awareness, Plato explored ideal forms and the philosopher-king concept, and Aristotle laid the groundwork for logic and empirical observation. Philosophy flourished across diverse regions and eras after that. Medieval thinkers grappled with religious themes, while the Renaissance saw a revival of classical works. Enlightenment philosophers like Kant and Locke championed reason and individual rights, leading to further philosophical exploration in the 19th and 20th centuries.

Existentialism explored individual freedom and responsibility (Sartre, Camus), phenomenology delved into the nature of experience (Husserl), and logic and language analysis gained prominence through Russell and Wittgenstein. Feminism, critical theory, and postcolonialism emerged to challenge traditional narratives of knowledge and power.

Today, philosophy remains a vibrant field engaging with pressing issues across disciplines, from consciousness and artificial intelligence to bioethics and environmentalism.

Key Themes of Philosophy:
- **Metaphysics:** Examining the nature of reality, existence, and the cosmos.

- **Epistemology:** Exploring the nature and limits of knowledge and how it is acquired and justified.

- **Ethics:** Delving into moral questions, exploring concepts like right and wrong, good and bad.

- **Logic:** Analyzing reasoning, argumentation, and the validity of conclusions.

- **Aesthetics:** Investigating the nature of beauty, art, and aesthetic experience.

- **Political Philosophy:** Considering the nature of justice, power, and the ideal society.

Philosophy's value lies not in providing answers but fostering critical thinking, intellectual curiosity, and challenging assumptions. It equips us with tools to analyze arguments, navigate complex issues, and form well-reasoned opinions.

As one delves into philosophy, remember that it is not a destination but a journey of exploration and self-discovery! Embrace the questions, revel in the complexities, and allow yourself to be transformed by the power of philosophical inquiry!

(Note: This overview is condensed and avoids technical jargon to provide a broad understanding.)

UNEARTHING WISDOM IN THE MODERN AGE: MELDING ANCIENT PHILOSOPHIES WITH CONTEMPORARY REALITY

As humanity forges ahead, a longing arises to reconnect with timeless wisdom lost amidst the hustle of modern life. Ancient philosophies like Stoicism, Buddhism, and Hermeticism offer enduring insights. Though distinct, they share resilience and practicality in navigating life's complexities. Stoicism emphasizes duty and the control of the controllable, Buddhism seeks enlightenment, and Hermeticism pursues esoteric knowledge.

- **The Blueprint for a Virtuous Life:** Central to these philosophies is the injunction to "know thyself." Understanding one's nature, motives, and triggers lays the groundwork for virtuous living. Emulating Stoic figures like Marcus Aurelius and Epictetus could lead to a life of resilience and tranquility.

- **Detachment in the Face of Uncertainty:** Non-reaction, the ability to respond rather than react, offers solace in today's noisy world. This momentary detachment enables composure in adversity and clarity amidst confusion.

- **The Power of Silence and Solitude:** Silence and solitude, often overlooked in a world of noise, facilitate introspection and inner wisdom. In solitude, one engages in a dialogue with the self, unearthing insights unavailable amidst life's clamor.

- **The Journey of Self-Cure: Reclaiming Our Shared Humanity:** Ancient philosophies advocate a holistic approach to healing the human spirit. The cure entails self-awareness and transformation, addressing the imbalance that permeates our lives.

- **Embracing the Shadows:** Plato's allegory of the cave urges introspection, confronting our fears and prejudices. Disillusionment with the shadows of our consciousness is a precursor to enlightenment.

- **Activating Inner Excellence:** Historical figures like da Vinci, Tesla, and Gandhi exemplify inner excellence through self-discipline and moral integrity. Their subtle and grand victories underscore the significance of personal growth.

In integrating ancient wisdom with contemporary reality, we embark on a journey towards self-discovery and collective flourishing.

CHAPTER 9

GLOBAL PEACE THROUGH PERSONAL REFORMATION

Pursuing global peace often begins with personal transformation, exemplified by historical figures like Socrates, Leonardo Da Vinci, Nikola Tesla, Harriet Tubman, and Buddha. Through their unwavering courage and integrity, they became champions for a world free from injustice and suffering, illustrating the profound impact of individual conscientiousness on societal consciousness.

Ancient Philosophers as Modern-Day Guides

Ancient philosophers continue to illuminate the path for present-day seekers. Their timeless teachings offer remedies for modern afflictions such as anxiety, restlessness, and alienation. By integrating their wisdom into our daily lives, we bridge the gap between antiquity and the contemporary world, tapping into a perennial source of guidance.

Learning from Greatness

The biographies of these luminaries serve as living manuscripts that chronicle the art of living. Their lives teach us about the boundless potential of humanity, the connection between creativity and order, and the transformative power of cultivating the mind.

Legacy and Continuity

The legacy we inherit is a matter of personal choice. As custodians of an unbroken chain of human aspiration, we carry the torch of knowledge. The convergence of ancient wisdom and modernity holds the promise of a civilization where the timeless truths of the past color futuristic dreams.

Embracing the Infinite

Driven by wisdom, the pursuit of knowledge and self-discovery propels us toward the boundless embrace of the infinite. This quest transcends temporal and spatial constraints, uniting diverse souls in pursuing enlightenment. As we navigate life's labyrinthine passages, let us carry the torch of ancient philosophies – Stoicism, Buddhism, Hermeticism – lighting our path and igniting the flames of personal evolution!

In Conclusion

Integrating ancient philosophies into modern life is not a nostalgic indulgence but an urgent call to harness collective wisdom for the challenges ahead. By echoing the words and wisdom of antiquity, we uncover a treasure trove capable of enriching our lives today and every day after that.

"The object of life is not to be on the side of the majority, but to be on the side of the truth." - Marcus Aurelius.

CHAPTER 10

STOICISM & MINDSET: A FELLOW TRAVELER'S CALL ON THE STOIC PATH
"A Note from Marcos Rodrigues Lorenzi"

By sharing personal experiences with Stoicism, the author invites readers to explore this philosophy and its potential to enrich their lives.

As you embark on this journey into Stoicism, a philosophy that has profoundly influenced the author's life, I offer a friendly note before we proceed. Stoicism isn't a shortcut to material wealth or personal glory; it's a potent tool for self-discovery, ethical living, and fostering resilient communities. However, in today's age, there's a concerning trend of misrepresentation, portraying Stoicism as a quick fix for worldly problems. Let's embark on this journey together, guided by clarity and open-mindedness! Here's my message to you:

1. **Own Your Learning!** Seek diverse perspectives, engage in critical thinking, and explore the works of esteemed Stoic philosophers! Proper understanding arises from active inquiry, not passive acceptance.

2. **Resist the Quick Fix Trap!** Stoicism isn't a magic solution. Lasting change demands consistent effort, introspection, and dedication. Avoid the allure of instant gratification; embrace the journey of self-development, one mindful step at a time!

3. **Protect the Integrity of Stoicism!** Stoicism isn't about personal gain or empty boasts. It's about cultivating virtue, living ethically, and contributing positively to society. Let's safeguard against misinterpretations and uphold the essence of Stoicism!

My Commitment to You

- **A Fellow Traveler, Not a Guide:** Like you, I'm on a lifelong journey of learning and exploration. Stoicism has been a profound source of wisdom for me, one I'm eager to share rather than dictate. This book is an invitation, not a roadmap.

- **We Walk Different Paths:** We all perceive the world differently, with distinct priorities and pursuits. That's perfectly natural. This book aims to spark curiosity about Stoicism and align with your journey.

- **Patience Is Key:** Authentic transformation unfolds over time. Forcing insights upon unwilling minds only breeds resistance. Let's approach this journey with patience and openness to new possibilities!

CHAPTER 11

MINDFULNESS PRESENT-MOMENT JOURNEY

Few concepts offer as soothing a respite within the bustling marketplace of human experience as mindfulness. Yet, beyond the popularized image of serene individuals meditating in lotus poses lies a multifaceted phenomenon worthy of deeper exploration. Like sunlight filtering through a prism, mindfulness refracts into various facets, each illuminating a unique aspect of our present-moment awareness.

HISTORICAL BACKGROUND OF MINDFULNESS

The concept of mindfulness has ancient roots, dating back thousands of years to Eastern contemplative traditions such as Buddhism. In Buddhist teachings, mindfulness is considered an essential element of the path to enlightenment. Early Buddhist texts describe mindfulness as watching the mind with detached awareness, observing its thoughts and emotions without judgment.

The mindfulness practice has spread from India to other parts of Asia, including China and Japan. In China, it became known as "mindfulness meditation" (chán zuò) and was incorporated into Taoist practices. It became known as "zazen" in Japan and was integrated into Zen Buddhism. In the 20th century, mindfulness began to gain interest in the West. Pioneering figures such as Thich Nhat Hanh and Hanh Dzũn Nguyên introduced mindfulness practices to Western audiences. In the 1970s, Jon Kabat-Zinn developed Mindfulness-Based Stress Reduction (MBSR), a program that combines mindfulness meditation with yoga postures and gentle movement. MBSR is effective in reducing stress, anxiety, and depression.

Since then, mindfulness has become increasingly popular in the West and used in various settings, including schools, hospitals, and workplaces. A growing body of research supports its benefits for mental and physical health.

THE SEEDS OF INSIGHTFUL BEING
The roots of mindfulness can be traced back to ancient Eastern philosophical and spiritual traditions, notably Buddhism. Central to these traditions is sati, or mindful attention, which means focusing on the present moment without judgment. Over time, mindfulness practices have migrated and evolved, finding resonance in diverse contexts, from healthcare and education to workplace settings and personal well-being.

BEYOND STEREOTYPES' VEIL
While often associated with meditation techniques, mindfulness encompasses a broader spectrum of practices and experiences. It's not merely about achieving a state of perfect mental stillness but rather about cultivating an awareness of our internal and external world with an open and accepting attitude. Imagine a gentle observer within you, witnessing thoughts, emotions, and sensations without being swept away by them!

CHAPTER 12

THROUGH THE KALEIDOSCOPE OF DIMENSIONS

Scholars exploring mindfulness highlight several key dimensions:

- **Attention:** Cultivating focused awareness on the present moment, directing attention to specific objects of experience, such as the breath or bodily sensations.

- **Acceptance:** Approaching thoughts, emotions, and experiences with a non-judgmental stance, observing them without getting caught up in their narratives.

- **Openness:** Cultivating a receptive and curious mind, allowing experiences to unfold without resistance or preconceived notions.

- **Awareness:** Encompassing bodily sensations, emotions, thoughts, and external stimuli, fostering a sense of interconnectedness with the present moment.

IMPLICATIONS FOR THE INQUISITIVE MIND

Understanding the multifaceted nature of mindfulness opens doors to diverse applications and benefits:

- **Stress Reduction:** Cultivating present-moment awareness can interrupt patterns of worry and rumination, fostering a sense of calm and greater emotional resilience.

- **Enhanced Attention and Focus:** Mindfulness practices can improve cognitive functioning, leading to better concentration, reduced distractibility, and increased productivity.

- **Self-Compassion and Acceptance:** Mindfulness can foster self-compassion and acceptance by observing thoughts and emotions with detachment, leading to a more forgiving relationship with oneself.

- **Improved Relationships:** Mindfulness practices can enhance communication and empathy, fostering deeper connections with others.

AN ONGOING EXPLORATION

Mindfulness research continues to blossom, with ongoing investigations into:

- **Neuroscientific Foundations:** Exploring the neural correlates of mindfulness practice and examining how it impacts brain activity and cognitive processes.

- **Clinical Applications:** Investigating the efficacy of mindfulness-based interventions in treating various mental health conditions, such as anxiety and depression.

- **Mindfulness and Social Change:** Exploring the potential of mindfulness practices to foster compassion, empathy, and social justice initiatives.

Mindfulness is not a quick fix or a fleeting trend but a gateway to a more prosperous, more present-moment existence. By appreciating its multifaceted nature, cultivating its various dimensions, and integrating its practices into our daily lives, we can unlock doors to greater well-being, connection, and self-understanding. So, dear reader! Join me on this journey of mindful exploration! Let us awaken to the present moment, cultivate inner peace, and discover the transformative power of conscious beings! Remember! The present moment awaits an open invitation to pause, breathe, and be.

CHAPTER 13

MINDFULNESS PRACTICES TOOLBOX

Day 1: Anchor in Your Breath!
- **Practice:** Start with 5 minutes of mindful breathing! Sit comfortably, close your eyes (optional), and focus on your breath entering and leaving your nostrils. Notice the rise and fall of your chest and abdomen without judgment. When your mind wanders, gently bring your awareness back to your breath.

- **Impact:** These simple practices anchor you in the present moment, reducing stress and improving focus.

Day 2: Body Scan for Relaxation
- **Practice:** Lie down comfortably and do a mental body scan! Start with your toes and gradually move up, noticing any sensations without judgment. Are your toes tense or relaxed? Is your breath shallow or deep? Observe without judgment and release any tension you find.

- **Impact:** This practice cultivates body awareness and promotes relaxation, reducing anxiety and improving sleep.

Day 3: Mindful Eating
- **Practice:** Choose a small snack and eat it mindfully! Notice the colors, textures, smells, and tastes of each bite. Chew slowly and savor the experience. Pay attention to your hunger and fullness cues, stopping when satisfied.

- **Impact:** This practice improves your relationship with food, promotes healthy eating habits, and combats emotional eating.

Day 4: Gratitude List

- **Practice:** Before bed, list five things you are grateful for, big or small! Reflect on the positive aspects of your day and cultivate an attitude of appreciation.

- **Impact:** This practice cultivates positive emotions, reduces negativity, and improves overall well-being.

Day 5: Mindful Listening

- **Practice:** Engage in a conversation with someone, giving them your full attention! Listen actively without interrupting or thinking about what you want to say next. Focus on understanding their perspective and being present in the moment.

- **Impact:** This practice strengthens communication skills, fosters empathy, and deepens relationships.

Day 6: Observe Your Thoughts!

- **Practice:** Spend 5 minutes observing your thoughts without judgment. Acknowledge them as passing phenomena, like clouds in the sky. Please don't get caught up in their content or believe them true.

- **Impact:** This practice reduces the power of negative thought patterns, increases self-awareness, and enhances emotional regulation.

Day 7: Mindful Movement

- **Practice:** Take a mindful walk, focusing on your body sensations and environment! Notice how your feet touch the ground, the feeling of the sun or wind on your skin, and the sounds you hear.

- **Impact:** This practice combines physical activity with mindfulness, reducing stress, improving mood, and boosting energy levels.

Day 8: Loving-Kindness Meditation

- **Practice:** Start by wishing yourself well-being and happiness! Then, extend this intention to loved ones, acquaintances, and even neutral or challenging individuals. Repeat phrases like "May you be happy, may you be healthy, may you be peaceful!"

- **Impact:** This practice cultivates compassion, reduces negativity, and promotes inner peace.

Day 9: Accepting Imperfection

- **Practice:** Reflect on a situation where you felt inadequate or judged yourself harshly! Acknowledge your imperfections and remind yourself that everyone makes mistakes. Practice self-compassion and acceptance.

- **Impact:** This practice reduces self-criticism, increases self-esteem, and promotes emotional resilience.

Day 10: Limiting Screen Time

- **Practice:** Choose a specific time daily (e.g., 30 minutes) to disconnect from screens (phones, computers, TV)! Engage in activities that require your presence, such as reading, talking with loved ones, or hobbies you enjoy.

- **Impact:** This practice reduces digital distraction, increases mindfulness in daily life, and improves focus and concentration.

Day 11: Celebrate Victories (Big & Small)!

- **Practice:** Take time to acknowledge your big and small achievements and reflect on your progress. I appreciate your efforts! Celebrate wins with loved ones or indulge in a small reward.

- **Impact:** This practice reinforces positive behavior and motivates continued growth.

Day 12: Reflect & Integrate!

- **Practice:** Reflect on your mindfulness journey over the past 12 days! Consider how these practices have impacted your daily life and well-being. Integrate mindfulness into your routine, cultivating present-moment awareness and self-compassion.

- **Impact:** This reflection lets you consolidate your mindfulness practice and set intentions for continued growth and exploration.

QUOTES TO INSPIRE MINDFULNESS

- Buddha: "Holding on to anger is like drinking poison and expecting the other person to die."

- Lao Tzu: "The quieter you become, the more you can hear."

- Thich Nhat Hanh: "Mindfulness is the miracle that transforms your life into art."

- Ajahn Brahm: "Where can you go? You are already here. What can you do? You are already doing it."

These quotes underscore the essence of mindfulness, reminding us of the importance of present-moment awareness, acceptance, and inner peace.

CHAPTER 14

A SYMPHONY OF LIFE: EXPLORING THE MARVELS OF THE HUMAN BODY

"The human body is the greatest masterpiece of nature." - Michelangelo.

This quote beautifully captures the awe-inspiring complexity of the human body, a symphony of interconnected systems performing a delicate dance of life.

The Body as a Symphony: Exploring the Marvels of the Human Body

Shifting gears, we delve into the fascinating workings of the human body, appreciating it as a complex and interconnected system.

Imagine a magnificent clockwork, a universe contained within your skin! This intricate machine, the human body, comprises 11 distinct systems in a breathtaking symphony. From the circulatory system, pumping the lifeblood through our veins, to the nervous system, conducting the electrical orchestra of thought and action, each component plays a vital role in the grand performance.

But amidst the complexities of the modern world, how often do we genuinely pause to contemplate the marvel we inhabit? We readily engage in discourse, forming opinions on vast and intricate topics. Yet, can we confidently explain the complicated ballet of our digestion or the delicate dance orchestrated by the endocrine system? Perhaps it's time to embark on an inward voyage, a journey of self-discovery that begins not with the cosmos but with the intricate universe residing within. As we delve deeper into the unexplored territories of our bodies, a profound question emerges: If we are still unraveling the secrets of this intricate machine, how can we claim to understand the vastness of the outside world fully?

QUANTIFIABLE WONDERS: GLIMPSES INTO THE VASTNESS OF THE HUMAN BODY

Let's delve into some quantifiable wonders that make us who we are!

Cellular:

- Cells: Approximately 37.2 trillion (estimate varies based on methodology), each a tiny universe of bustling activity.

- Types of cells: Over 200 cells have been identified, each with specialized functions, from muscle contraction to nerve impulses.

- Gut bacteria: An estimated 100 trillion bacterial residents are crucial for digestion, immune function, and mood regulation.

Skeletal:

- Bones: 206 individual bones and a sturdy framework supporting our structure and movement.

- Joints: Over 360 synovial joints, allowing for flexibility and a wide range of motion.

Muscular:

- Skeletal muscles: Over 600 named engines power our every action, from blinking to sprinting.

Nervous:

- Neurons: There are approximately 86 billion in the brain alone, forming trillions of connections responsible for thought, emotion, and sensory perception.

- Length of the longest nerve: Sciatic nerve, approximately 4 ft (1.2m), carrying signals from the lower back to the foot.

Cardiovascular:

- Heartbeats per day: Approximately 100,000 (varies based on activity level), tirelessly pumping life-giving blood throughout the body.

- Total blood volume: Approximately 5 liters (varies by individual). Blood is a river of life that carries oxygen, nutrients, and waste products.

- The length of blood vessels is approximately 60,000 miles (96,560 km), a vast network delivering vital resources to every corner of our being.

Respiratory:

- Breaths per minute: 12-20 at rest (varies based on activity level), each inhalation a symphony of muscles and gas exchange, sustaining our very existence.

- Lung capacity: Approximately 6 liters (depending on the individual). The bellows fuel our internal fire.

Sensory:

- Taste buds: Approximately 10,000, painting a delicious map of flavors on our tongue.

- Olfactory receptors: Approximately 6 million, detecting a universe of scents and triggering memories and emotions.

Additional:

- DNA: Approximately 3 billion base pairs are in each cell nucleus, the blueprint of life passed down through generations.

- Air breathed per day: Approximately 11,000 liters, a testament to the tireless work of our lungs.

- The average lifespan is approximately 79 years globally (depending on region and other factors), a finite journey filled with countless possibilities.

Remember! These are just glimpses into the vastness of the human body. Each number represents an intricate system, each cell a world unto itself. As we explore these quantifiable aspects, let us also marvel at the unquantifiable: the resilience of the human spirit, the power of love and connection, and the boundless potential we hold within!

May this exploration empower you to appreciate the incredible gift of your own body, a symphony of life playing out in every breath, every beat, and every thought!

CHAPTER 15

A SYMPHONY OF PERCEPTION ON HOW DOES YOUR BRAIN CRAFT REALITY, SHAPE BELIEFS, AND CALL FOR INTROSPECTION?

The Overture: Sensational Doors to Inner Worlds
Our brains, marvels of evolution, are intricate orchestras where information cascades and converges. While often considered separate entities, our five senses are not isolated portals. They act as a unified sensory tapestry, weaving the raw threads of sensation into the rich fabric of our lived experience. Through sight, sound, touch, taste, and smell, the world floods our brains, triggering a cascading symphony of neuronal activity. But this symphony doesn't simply record external stimuli; it constructs our reality, shaping our memories and beliefs and even influencing our unconscious decision-making.

From Sensory Echoes to Memory Melodies: The Neural Canvas
Each sensory input sets in motion a complex sequence of events. Photons dance on the retina, sound waves resonate through the cochlea, and tactile sensations ripple across the skin. Neural circuits light up and transmit these signals to various brain regions, where they are interpreted, integrated, and imbued with meaning. This process of perception is not passive; it is an act of creation. Our brain's canvas is not blank but a living tapestry under perpetual construction.

The Illusion of Certainty: A Cognitive Mirage
Despite this remarkable feat of neural artistry, our sense of certainty in what we perceive is often an illusion—albeit a compelling one. We believe that what we see, hear, and feel accurately reflects objective reality. But the truth is far more complex. Our senses can be deceived, and our brains, ever the interpreters of raw data, are subject to biases, misconceptions, and outright delusions.

A Dance Of Biases And Beliefs

Why does our perception differ so significantly from person to person, even on matters of shared experience? The answer lies in the interplay of our neural architectures and our rich tapestry of personal experiences. Our beliefs color our perception more than we realize, shaping how we see the world. Whether it's the influence of culture, education, or personal history, no two observers perceive the same rainbow with identical hues.

Rethinking Reality: The Brain's Role in Constructing Truth

The brain constructs reality by weaving together the disparate threads of sensation and memory. This mental model isn't a mere reflection of the world "as it is" but a personal, predictive, and weighted model. Consider the phenomenon of optical illusions! These intriguing puzzles reveal the gap between perception and reality and demonstrate the brain's predisposition to fill in gaps and make assumptions.

Sensation, Memory, and Bias: The Trifecta of Truth Perception

Sensory inputs are fleeting, yet our memories linger and can alter our sense of what was. This interaction between perception, memory, and belief forms the cornerstone of constructing truth in our minds. It's a delicate dance that can lead to substantial disparities between our truths and the broader, measurable realities of the world.

THE INFLUENCE OF SOCIAL AND CULTURAL ECHO CHAMBERS

Our beliefs are not formed in a vacuum. The soil of our social and cultural environments nurtures them. In the age of echo chambers and social media, the brain's construction of reality is subject to unprecedented pressures. Our virtual realities, calibrated to reinforce our existing beliefs, can lead to a myopic worldview increasingly detached from the nuanced fabric of the world.

The Call for Introspection: Embracing the Uncertainty

Given the intricacies of perception and the malleability of belief, what tools do we possess to navigate the realm of constructed truths? Surprisingly, the answer lies within the symphony of our neural activities. By honing the skills of introspection, we can begin to unravel the complex web of biases and beliefs that shape our reality. This is not a call to skepticism or pessimism but to cultivate a healthy sense of epistemic humility.

Embracing Uncertainty: A Path to Personal Growth

When we embrace uncertainty, we open ourselves to new perspectives and insights. The admission that our constructed realities are fallible is not a weakness but a strength. It fosters a mindset of continual learning and personal growth. The self-assuredness that often comes with unwavering belief is replaced by a more fluid, adaptable form of cognition—one better equipped to navigate the dynamic seas of truth and falsehood.

Cultivating Curiosity: The Antidote to Belief Rigidity

One of the most potent antidotes to belief rigidity is curiosity. By cultivating a curious mind, we can untangle the knots of certainty that often accompany our beliefs. Curiosity encourages us to explore alternative viewpoints, to question our assumptions, and to engage in dialogue rather than debate. In doing so, we transform our constructed realities from rigid edifices to dynamic, evolving landscapes.

THE FUTURE OF TRUTH IN A DIGITAL AGE

In an era of abundant but often unvetted information, the future of truth hangs in the balance. The dissemination of misinformation and the erosion of trust have sown seeds of doubt in the public consciousness. As purveyors of information, we must uphold the sanctity of truth and foster an environment where critical thinking and evidence-based reasoning can thrive.

The Intersection of Technology and Cognition

Advancements in technology have given us unprecedented access to information but have also presented new challenges in discerning truth from fiction. From deep fakes to algorithmic biases, the digital age poses a formidable foe to our perception. As we march forward, we must remain vigilant and develop new cognitive tools to counter these threats.

Building a Community of Critical Thinkers

Many individuals need help safeguarding the truth. This task requires the collective effort of a community of critical thinkers. By cultivating such a community, we can create a bulwark against the tides of misinformation. Through education, discourse, and promoting scientific literacy, we can empower individuals to navigate the digital landscape with understanding and discernment.

Conclusion

The symphony of perception, the grand performance that unfolds within the confines of our skulls, is a never-ending overture. The ongoing act of creation shapes our reality, constructs our truths, and guides our beliefs. As we move through this world, let us do so with open minds, ready to challenge our perceptions and harmonize with life's changing tempo!

It is time to embrace the uncertainty and listen to the voices of doubt in the quietest corners of our minds. In these moments of introspection, we grow, refine our senses, and cultivate the courage to stand in the presence of our constructed realities and call them what they are: not the truth but our best approximation. And in this continual overture, let us be the conductors of our cognitive symphonies, leading with wisdom, authenticity, and a relentless pursuit of the melodic thread that binds us all!

Lorenzi R.Marcos

CHAPTER 16

UNLOCKING THE MIND-BODY CONNECTION
Neuroscience and Philosophy in Personal Development

THE SOCIAL SYMPHONY: UNVEILING THE NEUROCHEMISTRY OF BEHAVIOR

Moving beyond the individual, this chapter examines the intricate dance of neurochemical processes that influence our social behavior and interactions. In an age where self-improvement resources abound, it's worth exploring the roots of our quest for personal development. More profound than mere trends, the desire for growth and the pursuit of well-being are rooted in the fabric of human existential experiences. This exploration becomes even more prosperous when we consider the amalgamation of neuroscience and philosophy, two seemingly disparate fields that converge to offer profound insights into our approach to nutrition, fitness, mindset, and mindfulness. Through their synergy, we can decode the complexities of behavior change, addiction recovery, and sustainable personal development. In this expansive theme, we'll understand how these interconnected disciplines can transform individual lives and the mentality underpinning a collective spirit for a better, healthier, and fulfilled world.

THE NEUROPHILOSOPHICAL APPROACH TO DIET AND NUTRITION

Dietary habits, often rooted deeply in cultural and individual histories, manifest in complex relationships with the mind. But what role do neuroscience and philosophy play in understanding and changing these habits?

Understanding the 'Why' Behind Food Choices

Philosopher Will Durant's adage, "You are what you repeatedly do," underscores the power of habit. But habits are driven by a web of complex interactions in the brain that dictate our decision-making processes. The neuroscientific approach to diet and nutrition first seeks understanding food choice's cognitive and emotional drivers. Are our food preferences formed from genuine physiological needs, or are they products of emotional regulation, social constructs, or marketing?

The Ethics of Eating: A Philosophical Perspective

On the other hand, philosophy offers the realm of ethics to the dinner table. Concepts such as animal welfare, environmental sustainability, and the implications of our food choices on global equity bring a moral dimension to diet-related decisions. Confronting these ethical considerations through a philosophical lens primes us for mindful consumption and a deeper connection to the sustenance that fuels our bodies and minds.

APPLYING NEUROPHILOSOPHY TO CHANGE OUR RELATIONSHIP WITH FOOD

By synthesizing these frameworks, we can approach diet transformation holistically. Understanding the neurological underpinnings of habit formation empowers us to adjust our dietary patterns. At the same time, the moral framework facilitated by philosophy ignites a conscious revolution in our relationship with food.

THE MIND-BODY UNISON IN PHYSICAL FITNESS

Physical fitness is often categorized as a pursuit of the body but is intimately connected to the mind. Unraveling the neurophilosophical aspects of fitness can redefine our approaches to exercise.

Motivation: The Neuroscientific Riddle

Why do some individuals seem to effortlessly maintain an exercise regimen while others struggle to climb the treadmill? Here, neuroscience delves into the mechanisms behind motivation. Dopamine, commonly associated with the brain's reward system, plays a pivotal role in the motivational circuitry, often firing when we engage in pleasurable or goal-directed behaviors. How can we harness this neurochemical to cultivate the intrinsic drive to exercise regularly?

The Stoic Gymnasium: Philosophy and Fitness

Stoic philosophers like Epictetus advocated for an internal locus of control, teaching that our responses to external events are within our power. Such philosophical precepts find resonance in fitness, encouraging individuals to take charge of their physical well-being as an aspect of personal autonomy rather than an act of external compulsion. Can the wisdom of the Stoics inspire a paradigm shift in our approach to fitness, positioning it as an act of self-mastery?

Integrating Body and Mind through Exercise
By integrating neuroscientific findings and philosophical wisdom, we can reconceptualize our understanding of exercise as a harmonious expression of the mind-body union. Such a paradigm inherently promotes sustainable physical regimens that are not just endured but embraced as vital components of our holistic well-being.

CULTIVATING MINDSET AND MINDFULNESS THROUGH NEUROSCIENCE AND PHILOSOPHY

Our mindset and the degree of mindfulness we practice shape our experiences and interactions with the world. Here, we dissect the roles of neuroscience and philosophy in these foundational aspects of personal development.

The Plastic Brain: A Neurophilosophical Gem

Neuroplasticity, the brain's remarkable ability to reorganize itself by forming new neural connections, is a groundbreaking discovery marrying neurobiology with the philosophical concept of malleable human nature. How can we leverage neuroplasticity to foster a growth mindset that sees challenges as opportunities for growth and learning?

The Philosophy of Being Present

Rooted in ancient philosophical practices, mindfulness has experienced a renaissance in the neuroscientific spotlight for its demonstrable impact on well-being. Philosophy illuminates the ephemeral nature of perceived reality and the fallacy of past-future dichotomies by dissecting the concepts of time and consciousness. How can we apply these philosophical tenets to cultivate a truly present and mindful way of life?

Synchronizing the Self: Mindset, Mindfulness, and the Modern World

In a fast-paced modern society, the synergy of a resilient mindset and cultivated mindfulness is an anchor, providing stability in the face of life's storms. We can appreciate the dynamic interplay between thought patterns, neurobiology, and subjective experience through the interdisciplinary lens of neuroscience and philosophy, paving the way for a more conscious and fulfilling existence.

CHAPTER 17

OVERCOMING ADDICTIONS AND BUILDING SUSTAINABLE CHANGE

Addictions, whether to substances or behaviors, represent formidable obstacles to personal development. How can we employ neuroscience and philosophy to understand addiction and catalyze sustainable change?

The Addicted Brain: A Neurological Prison

Neurobiological studies have illuminated the brain's profound adaptations in response to addictive substances and behaviors, explaining the pervasive grip they can exert. By mapping the neurobiology of addiction, we unravel the mechanisms of tolerance, craving, and compulsive use, leading to a more nuanced understanding of the condition.

Freedom of the Will: The Philosophical Debate

The concept of free will lies at the heart of discussions on addiction and behavior change. Philosophical inquiries into determinism, the idea that all events, including human actions, are determined by causes external to the will, challenge our perceptions of agency. Is free will necessary for instigating change, or can we reconcile deterministic forces with personal autonomy?

The Path to Liberation: Breaking the Chains of Addiction

Drawing upon the insights of neuroscience and philosophy, we chart a course toward addiction recovery and sustainable behavior change. By leveraging the brain's capacity for adaptation and employing philosophical tools for introspection and self-awareness, individuals can transcend the cycle of addiction and forge new paths toward well-being.

A Unified Journey: Navigating Personal Development through Neurophilosophy

As we traverse the landscape of personal development, the fusion of neuroscience and philosophy serves as our compass, guiding us toward a deeper understanding of ourselves and our place in the world. By integrating these disciplines, we unlock the transformative potential of the mind-body connection, forging pathways to holistic well-being and authentic fulfillment. Together, let us embark on this unified journey, embracing the wisdom of the ages and the insights of modern science as we chart a course toward personal growth, resilience, and flourishing!

CHAPTER 18

NURTURING SUSTAINABLE PERSONAL GROWTH

Personal development is not just about setting and achieving goals; it's a continuous, sustainable growth journey. How can the confluence of neuroscience and philosophy guide us in this lifelong pursuit?

The Science of Habits: Small Changes, Big Impact

Neuroscientific investigations into habit formation and change reveal the power of small, consistent actions in reshaping our lives. By understanding the mechanisms governing habitual behaviors, we can implement micro-changes that lead to macro-shifts in our personal development trajectories.

Philosophy as the Navigation Tool in the Conquest of the Self

Philosophy serves as a compass for personal growth in its enduring endeavors to explore the fundamental questions of existence. It offers contemplative practices, ethical frameworks, and existential inquiries that can inform our decisions and inspire us to live intentionally and authentically.

Sustainable Development in a Neurophilosophical Paradigm

Integrating these insights unearths the potential for a holistic, sustainable approach to personal development. The synergistic applications of neuroscience and philosophy can create a framework that catalyzes change and anchors it in our deepest values and aspirations.

In conclusion, the intersection of neuroscience and philosophy provides a rich tapestry of perspectives to enrich our approach to nutrition, fitness, mindset, and mindfulness. By engaging with these disciplines, we don't just upgrade our operating systems; we contribute to a more informed and conscious collective consciousness primed for lasting change and well-being.

Embracing these neurophilosophical underpinnings empowers us to nurture our development and contribute to a global ethos that values health, wisdom, and the sanctity of the human experience. Through this lens, we can indeed explore the bounds of personal growth and, in doing so, impact the world around us in profound ways.

CHAPTER 19

NEUROPLASTICITY

Neuroplasticity, often called brain plasticity, encompasses the dynamic nature of the brain's structure and function throughout life. This inherent property enables the brain to adapt, change, and reorganize itself in response to various stimuli, experiences, and injuries. Beyond the initial developmental period, neuroplasticity challenges the traditionally held view of the brain as a static organ, offering exciting possibilities for learning, recovery, and overall cognitive health.

Mechanisms of Change:
At the cellular level, neuroplasticity manifests through several vital mechanisms:

- **Neurogenesis**: Refers to generating new neurons, primarily in the hippocampus and olfactory bulb. Recent research confirms that adult neurogenesis plays a role in learning and memory formation.

- **Synaptic plasticity**: Focuses on the strengthening and weakening connections between existing neurons. Experiences can lead to Long-Term Potentiation (LTP), strengthening specific pathways through increased glutamate release and enhanced receptor activity. Conversely, Long-Term Depression (LTD) weakens connections deemed less relevant.

- **Myelination**: Myelin sheaths insulate neuronal axons, facilitating faster communication. New experiences can promote myelination in relevant pathways, enhancing information processing efficiency.

- **Neurovascular coupling**: Increased neuronal activity triggers changes in local blood flow, ensuring adequate oxygen and nutrient supply to support plasticity-related processes.

Modulators of Neuroplasticity:
Numerous factors influence the extent and effectiveness of neuroplasticity:

- **Age**: While adult neurogenesis declines, other forms of plasticity, like synaptic consolidation, remain robust even in elderly individuals.

- **Genetics**: Variations in genes related to neurotransmission and neuronal growth can influence individual differences in plastic potential.

- **Environmental factors**: Stimulating environments rich in learning opportunities, physical activity, and social interaction promote enhanced plasticity. Conversely, stress, neglect, and sensory deprivation can hinder it.

- **Neurotransmitters**: Brain chemicals like dopamine, serotonin, and BDNF (Brain-Derived Neurotrophic Factor) play crucial roles in orchestrating and regulating plasticity-related processes.

Applications and Implications:
Understanding neuroplasticity holds immense potential for various fields:

- **Cognitive enhancement**: Brain training programs, cognitive-behavioral therapy, and mindfulness practices leverage plasticity to improve memory, attention, and executive function.

- **Rehabilitation**: After the stroke, injury, or neurodegenerative diseases, targeted interventions aim to rewire or re-establish lost neural connections, promoting functional recovery.

- **Mental health**: Neuroplasticity-based techniques are explored for treating depression, anxiety, and addiction by addressing maladaptive cognitive patterns and fostering healthier neural pathways.

THE BRAIN BEHIND THE CHANGE: A HISTORICAL JOURNEY THROUGH NEUROPLASTICITY

Imagine your brain not as a rigid, unchanging organ but as a dynamic landscape, constantly rewiring and remodeling based on your experiences. This fascinating ability, known as neuroplasticity, has sparked the curiosity of scientists for centuries, and its implications continue to revolutionize our understanding of learning, recovery, and the very nature of ourselves.

The seeds of neuroplasticity research were sown as early as the 19th century. In 1890, American psychologist William James proposed the idea of the brain as a "plastic" organ, adaptable to new information and experiences. However, the term "neuroplasticity" did not appear until 1948, when Polish neuroscientist Jerzy Konorski coined it. His work and studies by Spanish anatomist Santiago Ramón y Cajal challenged the belief that the brain was fixed after childhood, paving the way for further exploration.

The mid-20th century saw significant advancements. In 1961, Canadian psychologist Donald Hebb introduced his Hebbian theory, stating that "neurons that fire together wire together." This groundbreaking concept explained how repeated stimulation strengthens connections between neurons, forming the basis of our understanding of learning and memory.

Further evidence poured in throughout the following decades. Studies by American neuroscientist Michael Merzenich on monkeys revealed that cortical maps could reorganize after sensory deprivation, highlighting the brain's ability to adapt even in adulthood. Similarly, work by Swedish neuroscientist Eric Kandel on memory in sea slugs demonstrated the molecular mechanisms underlying synaptic plasticity, earning him a Nobel Prize in 2000.

Today, research continues to unlock the secrets of neuroplasticity. Studies using imaging techniques like fMRI allow us to visualize changes in brain activity in real time as individuals learn new skills or recover from injuries. Additionally, identifying genes influencing plasticity paves the way for personalized interventions to maximize its potential.

Lorenzi R.Marcos

CHAPTER 20

THE SCIENCE OF GROWTH, NEUROPLASTICITY, AND MINDSET

As we stand at the precipice of discoveries, the history of neuroplasticity is a testament to the brain's remarkable potential for change. By delving deeper into its mechanisms and harnessing its power, we open doors to a future where learning has no limits, recovery is a reality, and our understanding of ourselves expands beyond ever-imagined boundaries.

Interested in Further Exploration?

- **A History of the Concept of Neuroplasticity:** Read more

- **Hebbian Theory:** Learn more

- **The Molecular Basis of Learning and Memory:** Dive in

- **Learning to See: Lessons from the Owl:** Watch now

- **Beyond the Individual:** Acknowledging the Power of Neuroplasticity

While acknowledging each individual's unique journey, this chapter introduces the concept of neuroplasticity, highlighting the brain's remarkable potential for change.

BEYOND THE BUZZ: UNVEILING THE NEUROCHEMISTRY OF SOCIAL BEHAVIOR (AND WHY JUDGING IS NOT THE ANSWER)

Have you ever wondered why a colleague becomes the life of the party after a few drinks? Or why someone struggling with sugar cravings seems more irritable than usual? The answer lies in their choices and the intricate dance of neurochemicals within their brains.

Dopamine, the pleasure maestro, gets a standing ovation from substances like alcohol, nicotine, and even sugar in excess. This neurochemical reward system is why we crave those feel-good moments, potentially leading to repetitive behaviors. But before we point fingers, let's delve deeper.

Serotonin, the mood modulator, also joins the party with some of these substances, impacting impulsivity and social interactions. Imagine someone struggling with low serotonin! They might appear withdrawn or easily agitated, leading to misinterpretations and judgments.

Glutamate, the brain's energizer, gets a jolt from cocaine and some synthetic drugs, altering alertness and cognition. This can manifest as erratic behavior, but attributing it solely to the substance ignores the potential underlying issues that might be driving its use.

The truth is that the brain's chemistry is a complex web, and attributing social behaviors solely to substance use is like judging a book by its cover. Genetics, personality, past experiences, and social context all play crucial roles.

So, the next time you see someone engaging in seemingly unusual social behavior, remember:

- Judging is not the answer. It fuels stigma and hinders understanding.

- Seek to understand, not condemn. Consider the various factors that might be at play!

- Empathy is the key. Imagine their struggles, unique brain chemistry, and the social pressures they might face!

Lorenzi R.Marcos

Let's spark meaningful conversations instead of gossiping or engaging in small talk! Ask open-ended questions, listen actively, and offer support without judgment! Remember! Substance use is often a symptom, not the root cause.

This is a call to self-awareness. Let's educate ourselves about the complexities of brain chemistry and social behavior, move beyond snap judgments, and embrace empathy! We can create a more understanding and supportive world one conversation at a time.

Remember! The brain is a fascinating mystery, and judging individuals based solely on their choices is like feeling a wave for its crash without understanding the vast ocean beneath. Let's dive deeper together!

CHAPTER 21

THE MARKETING PYRAMID: HEALTH - WEALTH - RELATIONSHIP

We are the target because Adenosine triphosphate (ATP) is the energy currency of cells and is used for various cellular processes. Although it is not known who may have been the very first to utter this phrase, or some version of it, the earliest readily identifiable use of the word was by Jean Anthelme Brillat-Savarin in 1826, in his seven-volume book "The Physiology of Taste." He wrote, "Tell me what you eat, and I will tell you what you are."

We are nourished by what we feed ourselves, not just on our plates but also our minds and hearts. The sights and sounds we consume shape our perspectives, and the stories we tell ourselves define our possibilities.

A Neurophilosophical Perspective

In a world as complex as ours, laden with the lures of commerce and the tactile intricacies of existence, there is a continuous battle for our attention and, more intricately, our being. In vehement opposition to the marketing pyramid that schematically orders our interests, I delve into a neurophilosophical argument urging humanity to redefine its priorities according to a more profound understanding of human nature, purpose, and potential.

The Pristine Slate of Birth

At our genesis, we are pristine beings devoid of the mental clutter that encumbers cognizance in the journey ahead. This purity is embodied in a state of contentment, a semblance of happiness untainted by the consumerist ideals we're systematically spoon-fed. The neuroscientific implications are profound since they suggest a natural propensity towards well-being compromised over time by materialistic aspirations and a societal framework that tacitly encourages it.

The Inner Gears of the Human Mind
The fusion of neuroscience with philosophy plays a guiding role in calibrating the human psyche. From the peculiarities of the human brain to the nature of consciousness, this union elucidates the cogent underpinnings of our cognitive and affective systems. Understanding the ebb and flow of neurochemicals that regulate our states of being – from dopamine's allure to serotonin's calm – is pivotal in unraveling the enigma of personal development.

Marketing as the Master Puppeteer
We are mere marionettes to marketing; our strings are pulled precisely, nudging us towards an existence where our wants often precede our actual needs. The stratification of goods, services, and experiences into a pyramid echoes the capitalist world's financial hierarchy. It is a carefully constructed web with enticements and pitfalls, striving to keep us obedient and forever under its influence.

Faith in Fitness, Nutrition, and Mindfulness
If we break free from this influence, the transformative trifecta of fitness, nutrition, and mindfulness will be our guiding lights. Each pillar is integral to our well-being, with fitness invigorating our physical fortitude, nutrition nourishing our inner sanctum, and mindfulness nurturing mental clarity. In this, the philosophy of self-enhancement through these tenets is not merely a pursuit but a responsibility that fortifies us against the whims of marketing and the mental slavery it perpetuates.

THE SEPARATION OF PROBLEMS INTO IN AND OUT-OF-CONTROL SPHERES

The stoic wisdom of categorizing problems into domains we can influence and those we cannot is particularly salient in this context. Our arrogance in differentiating between the two assures that we expend energy where it is most fruitful rather than futilely combating the intangibles. This discernment and a thoughtfully applied neurophilosophy steer our being into calmer, more self-aware waters.

Epictetus, Discourses, Book 4, Chapter 1: "Man is not worried by events themselves but by his views of them." This quote highlights that our reactions to external events, not the events themselves, determine our well-being. We can't control what happens, but we control how we interpret and respond to it.

"You have power over your mind – not outside events. Realize this, and you will find strength." (Book 12, Meditation 18) This highlights the core Stoic principle that what truly matters is not the external world but how you interpret and respond to it. Self-control empowers you to maintain inner peace even in challenging situations.

"Turn your desire into stone. Quench your appetites. Keep your mind centered on itself." (Book 7, Meditation 38) This quote emphasizes the importance of discipline and willpower in shaping your desires and actions.

"Waste no more time arguing about what a good man should be. Be one." (Book 10, Meditation 4) This quote encourages action and taking personal responsibility for your development rather than simply thinking about it. Marcus Aurelius (121-180 AD), Roman emperor (161-180 AD) and Stoic philosopher, wrote "Meditations."

The Interconnected Quest for Health, Wealth, and Relationships

The age-old health, wealth, and relationships trinity are perennially sought after. However, our approach to these pursuits often mirrors the tenets of the marketing pyramid—our quest for health inundated with fad diets, our pursuit of wealth with conspicuous consumption, and our endeavor for relationships with virtual social currency. It is imperative to scrutinize the authenticity of these pursuits, infusing them with the values that are uniquely ours.

Conclusion: An Authentic Path to Self-Realization

Steering clear of the marketing pyramid, we embark on a path to self-realization void of artificial benchmarks and fickle successes. It requires a departure from the mass-induced desires towards a customized voyage, mapped by our philosophy and anchored in the underlying principles of neuroscience. As we untangle the web spun by the puppeteer's alluring strings, our actions, diets, exercise regimes, and mental practices testify to our autonomy, discernment, and, ultimately, our freedom.

CHAPTER 22

EMBRACING NEUROPHILOSOPHY - A HOLISTIC APPROACH TO HUMAN WELL-BEING

In advocating for the principles of neurophilosophy, we do not dismiss the invaluable advancements of science; instead, we embrace them in a context deeply aligned with our primal essence. Within the delicate interplay of discipline, consciousness, and celebrating our holistic selves, we uncover our true calling — to become architects of our well-being uniquely humanly. Our journey toward liberation from the confines of the marketing paradigm is, therefore, a reclamation of what it means to lead a life imbued with intention, purpose, and fulfillment.

MINDSET: YOUR STALWART COMPANION ON LIFE'S ODYSSEY

Imagine your mind as a garden, where every seed planted — whether thoughts, beliefs, or expectations — burgeons and shapes the landscape of your existence! This garden, my dear friend, represents your mindset.

But what exactly is a mindset? It's not some esoteric concept beyond reach; instead, it's the fabric of how you perceive yourself, the world, and your capacity for growth and change. It's akin to that inner voice gently nudging you towards greatness or the pesky gremlin sowing seeds of doubt.

Nurturing a robust mindset is of paramount importance. Your mindset acts as a magnet, drawing experiences that mirror your beliefs. Think, "I lack financial prowess," and watch as opportunities for fiscal growth elude you. Yet, adopt the mantra, "I am mastering financial management," and behold, as avenues for prosperity unfurl before you.

Cultivating a resilient mindset mirrors tending to a flourishing garden. We desire bountiful plants, not pernicious weeds. So, how do we evade these treacherous traps in wealth, health, and relationships? Let's embark on this journey, starting with wealth! Picture "dark marketing" as those pesky pop-ups attempting to delight you. Their aim? Exploit your vulnerabilities and prompt unnecessary purchases. A sturdy mindset unveils these ploys, fostering discernment and mindful spending. It sows seeds of financial acumen, birthing a garden with prudent choices.

Health parallels this analogy. Bombarded by fad diets and unattainable fitness fads, we're akin to a garden besieged by weeds — enticing yet deleterious. A steadfast mindset fosters discernment, advocating for sustainable habits that nourish the body.

Your garden flourishes with vitality and well-being.

Relationships are akin to online scams that exploit trust and negativity corporate bonds. A fortified mindset acts as a beacon, illuminating toxic patterns and nurturing empathy. Your garden becomes a sanctuary of love and support through effective communication and healthy boundaries.

Yet, cultivating a robust mindset isn't effortless. It's akin to nurturing your garden — fraught with challenges like those unexpected weeds. But remember! This journey is one of progress, not perfection. Celebrate each victory, glean wisdom from setbacks, and never cease tending to your mindset! This is merely the genesis — let's delve into potent tools and techniques to nurture a mindset that empowers you to thrive in every facet of life!

MINDSET: REINVIGORATING YOUR CEREBRAL CIRCUITRY FOR TRIUMPH

Envision your brain as a labyrinth of intricate pathways, shaping your thoughts, emotions, and actions at every turn! This labyrinth, my friend, constitutes your mindset — the neural landscape where beliefs, expectations, and self-perceptions intertwine. But why delve into the intricacies of the brain? Your mindset isn't a nebulous concept; it's deeply entrenched within the physical connections of your brain cells. Every thought and experience fortifies some pathways while enfeebling others. This imparts upon you the power to sculpt your mental topography.

Picture a detrimental mindset as a thicket of tangled paths overrun by negative self-talk and constraining beliefs — akin to pernicious weeds hindering progress. Conversely, a resilient and optimistic mindset mirrors a meticulously tended garden, with clear pathways of optimism, resilience, and self-compassion. Such a mindset empowers you to navigate life's trials with poise, resourcefulness, and an indomitable spirit.

But how do we identify and extricate these mental weeds, nurturing a thriving mindset garden?

1. **Mindful Observation of Inner Dialogue**: Tune into your self-talk! Are you incessantly berating yourself or fixating on limitations? These are the weeds. Challenge negative thoughts, replacing them with affirmations that encourage you!

2. **Awareness of Emotional Responses**: Do fear and anger readily overwhelm you? These emotions often herald limiting beliefs; practice mindfulness and emotional regulation to navigate them adeptly!

3. **Analysis of Behavior**: Do you sabotage your success or procrastinate? Such behaviors typically stem from fear-based thinking. Identify the underlying beliefs and supplant them with strategies for action and fear mitigation!

4. **Embrace Neuroplasticity**: Your brain is in a perpetual state of rewiring! Engage in activities conducive to positive

thinking — from gratitude journaling to visualization and learning novel skills!

5. **Cultivate a Positive Environment**: Surround yourself with positivity — supportive relationships, uplifting content, or inspiring role models! Their buoyant energy enriches your mindset garden.

MINDSET: YOUR NEURAL ARCHITECT ERECTS INDOMITABLE PATHWAYS FOR ENDURING TRANSFORMATION

Visualize your thoughts, beliefs, and self-perceptions, weaving intricate neural highways throughout your brain! My dear friend, this interconnected network constitutes the essence of your mindset — shaping your experiences and long-term well-being.

But how does this nexus between mindset and neurobiology manifest?

- **The Synaptic Symphony**: Each thought, perception, and experience sculpts your brain's neural architecture through neuroplasticity. Consistent patterns of thought reinforce specific pathways while neglecting others. This affords your brain adaptability and learning prowess but renders it vulnerable to the pitfalls of negative mindsets.

- **Identifying the Weeds**: Consider the harmful impact of a poor mindset from a neurobiological lens. Rumination about negativity activates the amygdala — the fear center — triggering a cascade of stress hormones. Chronic stress enfeebles the hippocampus, impairing memory and learning. Furthermore, negative self-talk perpetuates a cycle of hopelessness in the brain.

- **Cultivating the Garden**: Conversely, a positive and resilient mindset fosters neural connections conducive to well-being. Practices like gratitude stimulate the reward center, releasing dopamine and kindling motivation. Learning new skills fortifies the prefrontal cortex, enhancing cognitive prowess. Mindfulness cultivates self-awareness and emotional regulation, activating the insula.

- **Beyond the Brain**: Mindset's ramifications extend beyond the neural realm, permeating physical and emotional well-being. Studies reveal that a positive mindset fortifies immune function, accelerates recovery, and augments longevity. Conversely, chronic negativity precipitates inflammation, cardiovascular sicknesses, and mental health disorders.

Lorenzi R.Marcos

- **Fitness and Nutrition**: This mind-body symbiosis pervades fitness and nutrition. A growth mindset fosters exercise adherence and encourages healthful dietary choices. Conversely, a fixed mindset sabotages fitness goals and compromises nutritional decisions.

- **The Lifespan Equation**: The dividends of a robust mindset accrue over time, influencing not just immediate well-being but longevity. Research demonstrates that individuals harboring a positive outlook tend to lead longer and healthier lives — underscoring the profound impact of mindset on longevity.

CHAPTER 23

YOUR 12-DAY MINDSET RESET: A SHORT JOURNEY OF SELF-DISCOVERY

Prepare to embark on a 12-day self-exploration, crafting a persistent mindset! This expedition necessitates no elaborate apparatus—solely your curiosity and willingness to delve within. Remember, this is your bespoke experience; heed your body's cues and tailor it to your biases!

Days 1-3: Communion with Nature's Embrace

- **Connect:** Commence daily with a 15-minute tour amidst nature's bounty! Immerse yourself in its sights, sounds, and fragrances, and record your sensory encounters and attendant emotions.

- **Reflect:** Take 10 minutes of silent meditation in nature's sanctuary! Abide with your thoughts without judgment.

- **Express:** Dedicate 15 minutes to journaling. Pour forth your aspirations, apprehensions, and reveries, and let your pen serve as your confidant!

Days 4-6: Nurturing Body and Soul

- **Fuel Up:** Commence your day with a nutritious breakfast with fruits, vegetables, and whole grains! Arm yourself with wholesome snacks to stave off sugar-induced crashes.

- **Move Your Body:** Select a light exercise that invigorates you—walking, swimming, dancing, or cycling! Aim for at least 30 minutes daily, relishing the camaraderie of others or the solitude of yourself.

- **Explore New Frontiers:** Discover a wholesome hobby that beckons your focus and creativity! Engage in gardening, painting, musical pursuits, or DIY projects, reveling in the process and celebrating incremental progress!

Days 7-9: Delving into Self-Understanding

- **Silence Speaks:** Dedicate 30 minutes to mindful silence! Retreat to a tranquil space, shut your eyes, and be attuned to ambient sounds! Witness your thoughts sans judgment, allowing tranquility to envelop your mind.

- **Gratitude Blooms:** Before retiring for the night, inscribe in your journal three gratitudes—cherishing life's minutiae and blessings! Nurturing gratitude begets a sunnier outlook.

- **Journaling Journey:** Traverse diverse journaling prompts each day. Contemplate your strengths, confront challenges, or chase dreams! This introspective voyage unveils the depths of self-awareness.

Days 10-12: Assimilation and Jubilation

- **Connecting the Dots:** Allocate time to peruse your journal entries from recent days! Discern patterns, emergent themes, or shifts in perspective! How has your mindset metamorphosed?

- **Celebrate Milestones:** Reflect on your triumphs, regardless of their magnitude! Have you experimented with a novel recipe or discovered a newfound passion? Acknowledge and praise your endeavors!

- **Blueprint for Tomorrow:** Drawing from your experiences, chart a course forward! What mindset practices will you perpetuate? What novel habits or hobbies will you assimilate? Devise a sustainable blueprint for the future.

Recall: This is only a suggested roadmap. Feel free to tailor the activities, duration, and pace to your preferences! Listen to your body, embrace curiosity, and relish the expedition of self-revelation!

Tips:

- **Share Your Odyssey:** Discuss your journey with a supportive confidant or family member!

- **Seek Inspiration:** Derive inspiration from online communities or mindfulness apps!

- **Courageous Exploration:** Don't discourage experimentation; explore diverse practices!

- **Cherish Every Step:** Celebrate each stride on your voyage, no matter how tiny!

With an open heart and a zest for exploration, you can cultivate a robust and empowering mindset that propels you toward triumph in every facet of existence.

CHAPTER 24

12 EXAMPLES OF A STRONG MINDSET: EMPOWERING YOURSELF AND THE WORLD

"Waste no more time arguing what a good man should be. Be one." - Marcus Aurelius.

MICRO AND MACRO BENEFITS OF A STRONG MINDSET

Wealth: From Scarcity to Abundance (Micro):
- **Shift:** Reformulate negative money dialogue. "I can't afford it" morphs into "I'm choosing to save for this."

- **Benefit:** Alleviates stress, encourages mindful spending, and unlocks new opportunities.

- **Macro:** Contributes to a sustainable and equitable society by valuing experiences over material possessions.

Health: From Body Shame to Self-Compassion (Micro):
- **Shift:** Prioritize progress over perfection! "I'm working towards a healthier lifestyle" supplants "I'm not good enough."

- **Benefit:** Bolsters motivation, diminishes self-criticism, fosters enduring well-being.

- **Macro:** Advocates body positivity and inclusivity, challenging unrealistic beauty standards.

Relationships: From Fear to Vulnerability (Micro):
- **Shift:** Foster authentic and transparent communication, even amid adversity.

- **Benefit:** Deepens connections, nurtures trust, and fortifies bonds.

- **Macro:** Cultivates an empathetic, interconnected society, mitigating loneliness and isolation.

Decision-Making: From Impulsivity to Clarity (Micro):

- **Shift:** Reflect on consequences before action. "What are my options?" replaces "I need this now!"

- **Benefit:** Mitigates impulsive decisions, fosters prudence, and enhances self-discipline.

- **Macro:** Cultivates mindfulness and sustainability, endorsing responsible resource management.

Challenges: From Obstacles to Stepping Stones (Micro):

- **Shift:** View challenges as opportunities for growth. "This is tough, but I can learn from it."

- **Benefit:** Augments resilience, instills perseverance, and hones problem-solving acumen.

- **Macro:** Fosters adaptability and innovation, empowering individuals to surmount adversity.

Gratitude: From Comparison to Appreciation (Micro):

- **Shift:** Appreciate personal blessings instead of coveting others' possessions.

- **Benefit:** Mitigates envy, amplifies contentment, and engenders joy.

- **Macro:** Cultivates a more grateful and generous society, diminishing negativity and competition.

Focus: From Multitasking to Mindfulness (Micro):

- **Shift:** Immerse in the present moment, eschewing distractions. "I'm doing this one thing at a time, with full focus."

- **Benefit:** Reduces stress, enhances productivity, and enriches quality of life.

- **Macro:** Promotes a mindful and present society, minimizing distractions and fostering well-being.

Learning: From Fixed Mind to Growth Mindset (Micro):

- **Shift:** Embrace learning and embrace challenges! "I can learn and grow from this experience."

- **Benefit:** Kindles curiosity, fortifies confidence, and unlocks novel opportunities.

- **Macro:** Catalyzes adaptability and innovation, nurturing lifelong learning and personal evolution.

Acceptance: From Resistance to Flow (Micro):

- **Shift:** Acknowledge circumstances beyond control! "This is happening, and I can choose how I respond."

- **Benefit:** Mitigates stress, enhances emotional well-being, and fosters mental clarity.

- **Macro:** Promotes serenity and resilience, urging individuals to focus on manageable aspects.

Contribution: From Self-Centeredness to Service (Micro):

- **Shift:** Seek opportunities to aid others! "What can I do to make a positive impact?"

- **Benefit:** Foster's purpose, nurtures connection, and enhances self-esteem.

- **Macro:** Cultivates compassion and solidarity, inspiring individuals to contribute to the greater good.

Forgiveness: From Holding Grudges to Letting Go (Micro):

- **Shift:** Release animosity towards oneself and others! "Holding onto this anger harms me more than it helps."

- **Benefit:** Diminished negativity, facilitated emotional healing, and fostered inner peace.

- **Macro:** Cultivates forgiveness and understanding, diminishing conflict and fostering reconciliation.

Meaning: From Confusion to Purpose (Micro):

- **Shift:** Align actions with a broader purpose! "What impact do I want to have on the world?"

- **Benefit:** Fosters motivation, engenders fulfillment, and imbues life with meaning.

- **Macro:** Propels a purpose-driven and engaged society, encouraging individuals to contribute to a collective legacy.

Conclusion: Embodying these principles transforms personal well-being and catalyzes societal progress. By nurturing a robust mindset, individuals become architects of their destinies, empowering themselves and enriching the world around them.

CHAPTER 25

DEVELOPING A STRONG MINDSET: A LIFELONG JOURNEY

As we navigate the complexities of life, it's essential to recognize that developing a strong mindset is a journey, not a destination. Here are some additional strategies to continue nurturing and strengthening your mindset:

1. **Self-Reflection and Awareness:** Regularly reflect on your thoughts, beliefs, and behaviors. Cultivate self-awareness by observing how your mindset influences your actions and emotions. Identify areas for growth and improvement.

2. **Continuous Learning:** Embrace a growth mindset by seeking learning and personal development opportunities. Be open to acquiring new knowledge, skills, and perspectives. Challenge yourself to step out of your comfort zone and explore unfamiliar territory.

3. **Resilience and Adaptability:** Cultivate resilience in the face of adversity by reframing challenges as opportunities for growth. Develop adaptive coping strategies to navigate setbacks and obstacles effectively. Embrace change as a natural part of life and remain flexible.

4. **Self-Compassion and Forgiveness:** Practice self-compassion by treating yourself with kindness and understanding, especially during difficult times. Let go of self-criticism and perfectionism, and forgive yourself for past mistakes or failures. Extend compassion and forgiveness to others as well.

5. **Positive Mindset Habits:** Incorporate positive mindset habits into your daily routine, such as gratitude journaling, mindfulness meditation, visualization, and affirmations. These practices help cultivate optimism, resilience, and emotional well-being.

6. **Surround Yourself with Positivity:** Surround yourself with supportive and uplifting individuals who encourage your growth and well-being. Seek positive influences in your social circle, community, and media consumption. Limit exposure to negativity and toxic environments.

7. **Set Meaningful Goals:** Set clear and achievable goals that align with your values, passions, and aspirations. Break down larger goals into smaller, manageable steps and celebrate progress. Remind yourself of your purpose and vision to stay focused and motivated.

8. **Embrace Challenges as Opportunities:** Embrace challenges as opportunities for learning, growth, and self-discovery. Approach obstacles with curiosity and resilience, knowing overcoming them will strengthen your mindset and character. View failures as valuable lessons and stepping stones toward success.

9. **Practice Gratitude and Mindfulness:** Gratitude and mindfulness are powerful tools for cultivating a positive mindset. Take time to appreciate the present moment and the blessings in your life. Focus on what you have rather than what you lack, and savor the richness of each experience.

10. **Seek Support and Guidance:** When needed, don't hesitate to seek support and guidance from trusted mentors, coaches, or therapists. Share your struggles, fears, and aspirations with others who can offer empathy, insight, and encouragement. Remember, you're not alone on your journey.

By incorporating these strategies into your daily life, you can continue to nurture and strengthen your mindset, empowering yourself to overcome challenges, pursue your goals, and live a life of purpose and fulfillment. Remember that developing a solid mindset is an ongoing process that requires patience, perseverance, and self-compassion. Embrace the journey, celebrate your progress, and strive to become your best version.

UNSHACKLING YOUR POTENTIAL: EMBRACING YOUR TRUE PURPOSE

In a world often dictated by societal norms and economic pressures, the idea of living your true purpose can feel like an intangible illusion. Yet, history is lined with luminaries who defied convention, listened to their inner voice, and brought to life their unique contributions. Leonardo da Vinci and Nikola Tesla aren't mere anomalies; they inspire the silent torchbearers of talent who yearn to break free from the mold and shine.

The Iron Grip of Society: A Historical Perspective

For centuries, countless societal pressures and norms have dictated individuals' endeavors. Feudal systems, industrial revolutions, and modern corporate ladders have all contributed to crafting a society where conformity often tramples creativity. Those brave enough to challenge the system frequently faced ridicule, hardship, and sometimes even persecution.

Socioeconomic Structures: The Silent Drivers

The need for survival has continually shaped socioeconomic structures, leaving a legacy permeating each generation. These structures provide a safety net but often at the cost of personal fulfillment and growth. Today, the structures are veiled under a veneer of choice, but the choices presented remain carefully orchestrated within the limits of societal expectations.

The Cost of Conformity

While conformity provides a sense of security, it often comes at a steep price—the erosion of individuality. Talents go undiscovered, passions remain unexplored, and dreams dissolve into the mundane of everyday life. The toll on mental well-being is significant, as the human spirit yearns for expressions beyond the confines it willingly succumbs to.

Rekindling the Flame: Seeking Your True Calling

The first step toward breaking free from societal norms is often the most daunting — recognizing that there's more to life than the predetermined path for you. Understanding your true calling is akin to peeling back the layers of socially constructed identity to uncover the raw essence of who you are.

CHAPTER 26

THE JOURNEY OF SELF-DISCOVERY

Self-Discovery: An Intricate Journey

Self-discovery is an intricate journey that requires introspection, courage, and, most importantly, time. It involves breaking away from the clutter of everyday life to find spaces where thoughts can wander freely and crystallize into an understanding of what truly ignites the spirit.

Learning to Listen to Your Inner Voice

To uncover your true calling, you must learn to listen intently to your inner voice despite the cacophony of external expectations. When heeded, this internal compass guides you toward activities that fill you with an inexplicable sense of joy and purpose. This joy, often misconstrued as the product of leisure, holds the key to unlocking a fulfilling vocation.

The Cultivation of Passion

Once identified, passions require nurturing. They are the seeds from which purpose blooms. Engaging in deliberate practice, seeking mentorship, and expanding knowledge in your areas of interest are pivotal in transforming passion into expertise.

Embracing Your Purpose: The Path to Mastery

Once you've identified your true purpose, mastery and actualization begin. Mastery is not the exclusive domain of the chosen few but the result of deliberate effort expressed over time.

The 10,000-Hour Rule Revisited

Malcolm Gladwell's "10,000-Hour Rule" is a testament to the power of practice in achieving mastery. Dedicate yourself to your craft, immerse yourself in learning, and over time, what once seemed impossible becomes your new norm!

Overcoming the Doubters

Doubters and naysayers are an inevitable facet of the path to mastery. Learn to differentiate between constructive criticism and

Lorenzi R.Marcos

baseless negativity! Your journey is yours alone, and the only validation you require comes from within.

Cultivating Abundance: Health, Wealth, and Relationships

Embracing your true purpose is a holistic endeavor that extends beyond professional life. It encompasses health, wealth, and relationships, which, when cultivated with purpose, become the pillars that support a fulfilling existence.

Health: The Foundation of Purposeful Living

A sound mind in a healthy body is not a cliché but a cornerstone of living purposefully. Regular exercise, a balanced diet, and mindfulness sustain energy levels vital for pursuing your passions.

Wealth: Redefining Abundance

As traditionally defined, wealth often becomes the end goal, overshadowing purpose. Redefine wealth as the abundance that results from living your purpose, not just in financial terms, but in experiences and contributions to society!

Relationships: The Social Ecosystem

Nurture relationships that support and encourage your journey toward purpose! Surround yourself with like-minded individuals, seek mentors, and be a mentor in return! A thriving social ecosystem elevates your quest for purpose and brings shared endeavors that enrich the human experience to light.

The Modern Renaissance: A Paradigm of Possibility

As we stand on the precipice of a new era, where technological advancements unravel the fabric of traditional work, there is an opportunity for a modern renaissance. The individual is empowered like never before to sculpt a life that aligns with their passions and purpose.

Technological Enablers of Individualism

The digital age provides many tools and platforms that propound individual expression. Content creation, remote working, and instant connectivity dissolve the demographic barriers that once confined aspirations.

Fostering a Culture of Purpose

Organizations and communities that foster a culture of purpose are becoming the beacon for those seeking to break away from the norm. These environments recognize that purpose-driven individuals are not just assets but sources of innovation and inspiration.

Living Without Fear of Failure: The Ultimate Freedom

Freedom from the fear of failure liberates the human spirit. Embracing the inevitability of stumbles and setbacks is a precursor to living your true purpose. Each failure becomes a stepping stone, a lesson, and a testament to your unwavering pursuit of a life lived authentically.

The Imperative of Personal Choice

The call to embrace your true purpose is not an appeal to abandon all that is known, safe, and familiar. It is an invitation to examine life's canvas and decide whether the strokes you paint express your being or a depiction of societal expectations.

Ralph Waldo Emerson's words resonate profoundly in this context: "To be yourself in a world that is constantly trying to make you something else is the greatest accomplishment." Remember that life is not a rehearsal as you journey towards your purpose. There are no retakes, and the curtain will eventually fall. Make every scene count, and let the narrative be a testament to your undeterred pursuit of self-expression and fulfillment!

N1: FORK AND FIELD - FOOD AND I

"Let food be thy medicine and medicine be thy food." - Hippocrates, Greek

My story begins in the sun-baked earth beneath my bare feet, with the aroma of freshly tilled soil filling my lungs. In the heart of a vibrant countryside, food wasn't just sustenance; it was a symphony of colors, textures, and aromas, a ritual woven into the fabric of life.

But my tale takes a twist, for life led me on an extraordinary journey across six continents. From the sun-drenched vineyards of Italy to the lively street food stalls of Brazil, from the spice-laden delicacies of Turkey to the precision-crafted cheese platters of Switzerland, each new land unfolded a treasure trove of culinary secrets.

In the bustling markets of London, I marveled at the global melting pot, while the vast farmlands of the USA instilled in me a reverence for the earth's bounty. I discovered flavors, cultures, traditions, and stories with each bite.

Whether witnessing Nonna's skilled hands rolling out pasta or learning the art of churrasco from a Brazilian Gaucho, food became a bridge connecting hearts and fostering understanding. This wasn't just about satiating hunger; it was about celebrating the very essence of humanity, our shared connection to the earth and each other.

But amidst this delicious tapestry, I saw shadows: the limitations imposed by factory farms, the exploitation of resources, and the disconnect between people and their food. These shadows ignited a spark within me, a fire for change.

Inspired by the ingenuity of Leonardo da Vinci and the revolutionary spirit of Nikola Tesla, both renowned vegetarians, I committed myself to advocating for freedom of choice and the right to access healthy, sustainable food for all.

This book is an invitation, a journey through the world of food and its profound impact on our lives. Join me as we explore the rich history of human sustenance, delve into the intricacies of nutrition, and celebrate the diverse tapestry of culinary traditions.

Let's break down barriers, empower individuals, and champion a future where food nourishes our bodies, communities, and planet. So, dear reader, grab your metaphorical fork and join me on this adventure. Let the pages become your passport to a world where food is more than just fuel; it's a force for good, a catalyst for change, and a powerful tool for shaping a healthier, more equitable tomorrow. The stage is set, and the feast awaits. Die in, and savor the journey!

N2: THE HUMAN JOURNEY OF EATING

A Bite-Sized History

Imagine our early Homo sapiens ancestors tirelessly foraging for berries and hunting wild game. Food wasn't just sustenance; it was a gamble, a daily struggle for survival in a world of scarcity. This was the dawn of our relationship with food, a primal dance woven into the fabric of existence.

Then came the agricultural revolution, a game-changer around 12,000 years ago. We transitioned from nomadic hunters to settled farmers, cultivating crops and domesticating animals. Food became less of a lottery and more of a controlled system, leading to population growth and the rise of civilizations.

But abundance brought its challenges. Famines due to unpredictable weather or crop failures became a constant threat. Empires thrived and crumbled based on their ability to secure food for their people. The quest for reliable sustenance fueled exploration, leading to the discovery of new lands and diverse food cultures.

Fast forward to the Industrial Revolution, and food production went into overdrive. Mechanization, artificial fertilizers, and global trade networks led to an unprecedented abundance of food. Supermarkets replaced farms as our primary source of sustenance, and convenience became king.

However, this "food utopia" came at a cost. The industrialization of agriculture led to environmental degradation, soil depletion, and a disconnect between people and their food. Processed foods became staples laden with sugar, salt, and unhealthy fats.

Today, we stand at a crossroads. Obesity and malnutrition coexist, food waste is rampant, and climate change threatens global food security. Our challenges are complex, but understanding our historical relationship with food offers valuable insights.

A Bite Out of History: Climate Change, Poisoned Plates, and the Future of Food

Our historical journey through the human relationship with food has revealed fascinating insights into our struggles for survival, the impact of agricultural revolutions, and the challenges of modern abundance. However, this narrative takes a sobering turn as we consider the looming threats of climate change, food contamination, and unsustainable agricultural practices.

This global picture demands a comprehensive and robust international view:

Climate Change and Its Bite:

Imagine a world where rising temperatures disrupt crop yields, extreme weather events devastate farmland, and water scarcity cripples irrigation systems. This isn't science fiction; it's the harsh reality of climate change's impact on food production.

The Intergovernmental Panel on Climate Change (IPCC) warns that a two-degree °C rise in global temperatures could reduce global food production by up to 25%. This would result in millions facing hunger and malnutrition, particularly in vulnerable regions already struggling with food insecurity.

The impact goes beyond production. Climate change disrupts food distribution as extreme weather events damage infrastructure and transportation networks. Rising sea levels threaten coastal communities and agricultural land. The ripple effects are felt across borders, destabilizing food markets and exacerbating global food insecurity.

Furthermore, climate change alters nutritional needs. As temperatures rise, the human body requires more calories and fluids, yet extreme weather events and changing precipitation patterns can disrupt the production of essential micronutrients like vitamins and minerals. This can lead to malnutrition and health problems, particularly for children and pregnant women.

Poisoned Plates? Addressing the Contaminants:

Our historical transition to industrial agriculture brought convenience and abundance but raised concerns about food contamination. Pesticides that protect crops can leave harmful residues, potentially impacting human health and the environment. Industrial pollutants like heavy metals and antibiotics used in livestock farming can also find their way onto our plates.

These concerns are not just limited to developed nations. In developing countries, where regulations and monitoring systems are often weaker, the risks of food contamination are even higher. This raises critical questions about transparency and responsible sourcing. Consumers deserve to know where their food comes from, how it's produced, and what potential risks it may contain.

Supporting sustainable and responsible agricultural practices is crucial. Organic farming, integrated pest management (IPM), and responsible sourcing from trusted and transparent producers can help mitigate the risks of food contamination and protect our health and the environment.

Looking Forward: A Sustainable Feast for All:

Our challenges are complex, but understanding our historical and international context empowers us to build a better food future. We can move towards a more resilient, equitable, and sustainable food system by acknowledging the threats of climate change, food contamination, and unsustainable practices. This requires a multifaceted approach:

- Investing in climate-smart agriculture: It is crucial to develop crops resistant to drought and heat stress, improve water management systems, and support small-scale farmers.

- Empowering consumers Is Key to this. Education about responsible sourcing, advocacy for transparency in food labeling, and support for local and sustainable agriculture are essential.

- Promoting global collaboration: International cooperation is essential to address climate change, share best practices in sustainable agriculture, and ensure equitable access to nutritious food.

Our ancestors navigated food scarcity and abundance throughout history. Today, we face a different challenge: building a food system that nourishes a growing population, respects the environment, and ensures justice and equity for all. By learning from the past, acknowledging the present, and working together, we can create a future where food is not just a source of sustenance but a powerful symbol of hope, resilience, and shared humanity.

Further Reading:

- Intergovernmental Panel on Climate Change (IPCC) Special Report on Climate Change and Land: Link

- Food and Agriculture Organization of the United Nations (FAO) State of Food Security and Nutrition in the World 2023: Link

- World Health Organization (WHO) World Health Report 2023: Link

N3: FOOD ON OUR PLATES, CHAINS ON THEIR LIVES: ENDING MODERN FOOD SLAVERY

Imagine biting into a juicy mango or savoring a cup of coffee, unaware of the hidden human cost. Sadly, the fruits of our labor – and literal fruits on our tables – often come at the expense of modern food slavery. Millions toil in exploitative conditions, facing forced labor, debt bondage, and abuse throughout the food production chain. This dark reality demands a global response, and you have the power to be part of the solution.

A Global Chain of Injustice:

From cocoa farms in West Africa to fishing vessels in Southeast Asia, stories of exploitation echo across continents. Farmworkers endure grueling hours, meager wages, and dangerous working conditions, often denied fundamental rights and freedoms. Children are forced to abandon their education for backbreaking labor. This injustice isn't just a distant issue; it affects the food we consume daily.

The Call to Action:

Change starts with awareness. Educate yourself about the complexities of modern food slavery and the specific challenges faced in different regions. Dig deeper into the supply chains of the products you buy.

Empowering Your Fork:

1. Choose ethically sourced products: Look for certifications like Fair Trade, Rainforest Alliance, or B Corp that promote fair labor practices and environmental sustainability. Research brands committed to ethical sourcing and transparency.

2. Support local farmers markets: Connecting directly with producers allows you to ask questions about their practices and support fair wages for local communities.

3. Raise your voice: Advocate for legislation that tackles modern food slavery. Write to your elected officials, join campaigns, and spread awareness on social media.

4. Amplify the stories of the voiceless: Share documentaries, articles, and personal narratives that illuminate the issue. Support organizations working on the ground to eradicate modern food slavery.

Together, we can create a ripple effect: Your informed choices, voice, and actions contribute to a powerful wave of change. By holding producers and retailers accountable, we can build a food system that respects human dignity and ensures fair treatment for all. Remember, every bite carries a story. Let's rewrite it together, ensuring that food nourishes not just our bodies but also our humanity.

The Food Illusion: Decoding Marketing's Mind Games for a Healthier You

Have you ever felt hypnotized by a perfectly staged cheese pull advert or succumbed to the siren song of a "limited-time offer" on sugary cereals? You're not alone. The food industry wields a powerful arsenal of marketing mind games designed to exploit our cravings and nudge us towards unhealthy choices. But fear not—knowledge is your secret weapon!

Unmasking the Tricks:

- Emotional Manipulation: Adorable cartoon mascots, heartwarming family moments, and promises of happiness – these emotional triggers bypass our logic and tap into our desire for belonging and positive associations. Don't fall for the feel-good facade; focus on the actual nutritional value.

- Sensory Overload: Vibrant colors, catchy jingles, and strategically placed supermarket products bombard our senses, creating a subconscious connection between pleasure and unhealthy foods. Stay mindful, make a list, and avoid impulse purchases.

- Hidden Health Claims: "All-natural," "low-fat," and "sugar-free" – these terms often mask unhealthy realities. Research ingredients, understand serving sizes, and don't be fooled by clever packaging.

- Portion Distortion: Supersized drinks, hidden sugars, and misleading serving sizes distort our perception of what constitutes a healthy portion. Read labels carefully, compare serving sizes, and prioritize whole, unprocessed foods.

- The Fear Factor: Fear of missing out (FOMO) and limited-time offers create a sense of urgency, pushing us to buy unhealthy options we might not usually choose. Stay calm, plan your meals, and not be pressured by artificial scarcity.

Empowering Your Choices:

- Become a Label Detective: Learn to decode food labels, understand ingredients, and identify hidden sugars and unhealthy fats. Knowledge is power!

- Plan Your Meals: Planning meals and snacks in advance helps you resist impulsive unhealthy choices throughout the day.

- Cook More at Home: Reconnect with the joy of cooking and the control it gives you over ingredients and portion sizes.

- Support Honest Brands: Seek companies committed to transparency, ethical sourcing, and healthy products. Your choices send a powerful message.

- Spread Awareness: Share information with friends and family, advocate for stricter regulations, and support campaigns promoting healthy eating habits.

Remember, you are not a passive consumer but an active decision-maker. By understanding the marketing tactics and making informed choices, you can break free from the food illusion and reclaim your health. Let your plate be a canvas for nourishing decisions, not a reflection of manipulative marketing.

Additional Resources:

- Access to Safe Food Initiative (SAFE)

- Food and Water Watch

- Environmental Working Group (EWG)

5 Recognized Global Institutions About Food Regulation:

1. World Health Organization (WHO)

   - Website: [Link]

   - Resource: Global Strategy on Diet, Physical Activity and Health: [Link]

   - Focus: Public health and promoting healthy diets are crucial to disease prevention.

2. Food and Agriculture Organization of the United Nations (FAO)

   - Website: [Link]

   - Resource: Codex Alimentarius: [Link]

   - Focus: Setting international food safety standards and promoting sustainable food production practices.

3. Global Food Safety Partnership (GFSP)

   - Website: [Link]

   - Resource: Food Safety Information Network: [Link]

   - Focus: Collaborative platform for information sharing and capacity building on food safety issues.

4. International Food Safety Authorities Network (INFOSAN)

   - Website: [Link]

   - Resource: Global Foodborne Illness Outbreak Alert and Response Network (GFOIRN): [Link]

   - Focus: Rapid warning and response system for foodborne illness outbreaks.

5. Consumer Union (CU)

- Website: [Link]

- Resource: Food Safety and Sustainability Centre: [Link]

- Focus: Non-profit organization that tests and rates food products based on safety, quality, and sustainability.

N4: FROM GLOBE TROTTER TO FOOD SLEUTH: TRACKING FOR SUCCESS

Have you ever embarked on a whirlwind adventure across diverse countries, savoring unique flavors and immersing yourself in vibrant cultures? If so, you've likely collected a passport full of delicious memories – and maybe a few questions about how these culinary journeys impact your well-being. Here's where food tracking becomes your detective hat, helping you understand your body's unique map!

Just like navigating a new city, tracking your food intake empowers you to:

1. **Be a Mindful Explorer:** Remember those bustling spice markets you encountered on your travels? Tracking helps you recall the taste and the ingredients, portion sizes, and how you felt afterward. This mindfulness allows you to appreciate the impact of different foods from different places on your body.

2. **Decode the Menu of Your Health:** Ever felt sluggish after a vibrant meal in one country? Tracking can help decipher the connection between specific foods and your energy levels, sleep patterns, and overall well-being. You become a detective, uncovering which foods fuel your best you across different cuisines.

3. **Chart Your Nutritional Course:** Managing your health goals requires direction, just like navigating the bustling streets of unfamiliar cities. Tracking allows you to visualize your dietary patterns across different countries, identify areas for improvement, and set realistic goals. Whether incorporating more local vegetables into your diet or balancing your protein intake across diverse cuisines, tracking empowers you to chart a course toward a healthier you.

Now, let's explore your tracking toolbox:

1. **The Traditional Notebook:** Simple and familiar, pen and paper allow you to jot down meals, ingredients, and

emotions associated with eating. It's a personal journal of your food journey across different countries.

2. **Tech-Savvy Tracking Apps:** These apps offer sophisticated data analysis and goal-setting support, from calorie counters to macronutrient trackers. They're ideal for those who like their information readily available.

3. **Photo Food Diary:** Capture the dishes you enjoy and their context—a bustling market in one country, a shared meal with friends in another. Visual reminders can be powerful motivators and evoke positive memories of healthy choices globally.

Remember, consistency is key! Please choose a method that fits your lifestyle and stick with it for a few weeks to see patterns emerge. The beauty of tracking: it's not about restrictions but about self-discovery. As you track across different countries, you'll learn.

CHAPTER 28
N5: FOOD THROUGH TIME: A DELICIOUS JOURNEY OF THE BIZARRE AND WONDERFUL

Prepare to have your taste buds and minds tantalized, dear reader, for we embark on a whirlwind tour of food history's most curious corners! Buckle up as we unveil:

1. **The Royal Poopsmith:** Yes, you read that right. In Medieval Europe, a "Groom of the Stool" was responsible for the king's waste. But here's the twist: they also tasted the monarch's food beforehand, acting as human "poison detectors." Talk about a high-pressure (and potentially unpleasant) job!

2. **The Chocolate Conundrum:** In 16th-century Europe, chocolate was considered an aphrodisiac and sinful. Luckily, its reputation evolved, and today, it's a global love affair, though still shrouded in some "dark" mystique.

3. **The Fiery Feast:** Fire ants, anyone? In certain parts of South America, these insects are a delicacy, fried, and enjoyed for their citrusy flavor. Are you feeling adventurous? Perhaps an ant taco is in your future!

4. **The Viking's Bloody Beverage:** Sláinte! But hold your horses; Viking mead wasn't just honey wine. Some versions included blood, which was believed to enhance strength and courage. While it might not be for the faint of heart (or stomach), it paints a vivid picture of Viking culture.

5. **The Fish Sauce Frenzy:** Garum, a fermented fish sauce famous in ancient Rome, could cost more than gold. Its intense aroma might not have been everyone's cup of tea, but it was a prized ingredient, highlighting the diverse culinary tastes throughout history.

6. **The Coffee Enema Craze:** You read that right again. In the 18th century, coffee enemas were believed to cure everything from headaches to hangovers. Thankfully,

modern medicine has moved on, leaving this bizarre practice to the dusty annals of history.

7. **The Moon Milk Mystery:** Cleopatra, the legendary Egyptian queen, reportedly bathed in donkey milk, which is believed to keep her skin youthful. While the science might be questionable, it adds a unique twist to her iconic image.

From Fueling Factories to Folklore: Food, Revolution, and the Industrial Breakfast

The Industrial Revolution transformed not just landscapes and economies but also our plates. Let's delve into the surprising story of how food fueled this era of upheaval, focusing on the iconic British industrial breakfast and its lasting impact.

From Grain to Gears: The Rise of the Working-Class Diet

Before the 18th century, most laborers subsisted on simple fare like porridge or bread. But the demands of factory work necessitated a new kind of fuel. Enter the protein-packed breakfast:

- **Meat:** Bacon, sausages, and kippers became staples, providing sustained energy and a sense of "hearty" nourishment.

- **Eggs:** Cheap and readily available, they offered protein and essential nutrients.

- **Beans:** Baked beans, a source of fiber and protein, became a budget-friendly staple.

- **Bread:** Toast or fried bread provides carbohydrates for quick energy.

- **Tea:** Strong, milky tea fueled the day and offered a comforting ritual.

This high-protein, high-calorie breakfast became symbolic of the working class, symbolizing strength, endurance, and the ability to power through long hours of manual labor.

More Than Just Calories: The Social and Cultural Significance

The industrial breakfast wasn't just about sustenance; it held social and cultural importance:

- **Shared Experience:** Families would gather around the table, fostering a sense of unity and communal spirit before heading out to their respective factories.

- **Symbol of Status:** A substantial breakfast signified hard work and upward mobility, differentiating "proper" workers from the marginalized masses.

- **Fueling a Nation:** This breakfast sustained the workforce that drove Britain's economic engine, playing a crucial role in the success of the Industrial Revolution.

A Legacy Beyond the Factory Walls

The industrial breakfast's influence extends far beyond its historical context:

- **The "Full English Breakfast":** This modern iteration, encompassing the traditional elements, remains a popular tourist attraction and national dish.

- **Global Adoption:** Similar high-protein breakfasts became prevalent in other industrialized nations, shaping global food cultures.

- **Shifting Trends:** Today, concerns about health and convenience have led to breakfast diversification, but the industrial breakfast's legacy lives on.

Food for Thought

The story of the industrial breakfast reminds us that food is more than just sustenance; it's intricately woven into the fabric of our history, society, and even personal memories. Exploring past foodways allows us to understand better our plates, ourselves, and the world around us. So, the next time you enjoy a hearty breakfast, remember the hidden history within each bite. It's a legacy fueled by revolution, community, and the enduring power of food to shape our lives.

N6: GURUS AND MARKETING: THE MASTERS OF MANIPULATION

Fad diets thrive on manipulation. They exploit our insecurities with catchy slogans, cherry-picked testimonials, and fear-mongering tactics. "Detox cleanses" demonize essential food groups, while restrictive elimination diets leave you nutrient-deprived. Remember, no single food or gimmick holds the key to lasting health.

The Downside of the Quick Fix:

- Unsustainable Practices: Fad diets often promote restrictive and unrealistic rules, setting you up for yo-yo dieting and disordered eating.

- Nutrient Deficiencies: Eliminating entire food groups without proper planning can lead to vitamin and mineral deficiencies, impacting overall health.

- Ignoring Individual Needs: These "one-size-fits-all" approaches fail to consider your unique bioindividuality and health conditions.

- Focus on Appearance, not Well-being: The emphasis often shifts to aesthetics rather than promoting genuine health and sustainable lifestyle changes.

Empowering Yourself with Real Food Freedom: Ditch the quick fixes and embrace a sustainable, balanced approach to eating:

- Focus on whole, unprocessed foods: Prioritize fruits, vegetables, whole grains, lean proteins, and healthy fats.

- Listen to your body: Learn your hunger and fullness cues, and eat intuitively.

- Develop mindful eating practices: Savor your food, eat slowly, and avoid distractions.

- Seek guidance from qualified professionals: Registered dietitians and licensed nutritionists can provide personalized advice based on your unique needs.

Remember, proper health is a journey, not a destination. There's no magic bullet, no one-size-fits-all solution. Embrace the power of real food, prioritize mindful eating, and build a healthy relationship with food, free from manipulation and fad diet gimmicks. Hippocrates wisely said, "Let food be medicine and medicine be thy food." Nourish your body with wholesome foods, and watch your health flourish naturally. Together, let's build a community empowered by knowledge, free from the shackles of diet gurus and marketing ploys. The key to health lies not in quick fixes but in sustainable, mindful choices you make every day. Choose freedom, choose real food, choose you.

N7: THE DIGESTIVE SYMPHONY: AN ORCHESTRATED JOURNEY OF NUTRIENTS FROM MOUTH TO GUT

The human digestive system, a marvel of biological engineering, operates with the intricate coordination of multiple organs and processes. This "digestive symphony" begins when food enters the mouth and culminates in absorbing vital nutrients essential for life. Each stage is crucial in converting complex molecules into bioavailable components, influencing physical health and overall well-being.

The Overture: Mechanical Breakdown and Enzymatic Symphony The journey commences in the mouth, where food is physically fragmented by teeth and mixed with saliva. Salivary amylase initiates the chemical breakdown of carbohydrates, while other enzymes begin the digestion of proteins and fats. This orchestrated process, termed oral digestion, prepares the bolus for swallowing and further breakdown in the stomach.

The Oesophageal Interlude: A Muscular Passage Following chewing and swallowing, the bolus embarks on a brief but essential journey through the esophagus, a muscular tube lined with epithelial tissue. Rhythmic contractions, known as peristalsis, propel the food mass downward, aided by gravity. Sphincters at both ends of the esophagus ensure unidirectional flow, preventing reflux and protecting respiratory pathways.

The Stomach: A Powerful Mixing Vessel and Chemical Cauldron The stomach, a muscular sac-like organ, serves as the central processing unit of the digestive system. Powerful muscular contractions churn and mix the bolus with gastric juices, a potent cocktail of gastric acid, enzymes, and mucus. Gastric acid, with its low pH, denatures proteins and activates pepsin, an enzyme that further breaks down protein chains. The churning action facilitates the physical breakdown of food particles, increasing their surface area for enzymatic action. This phase, termed gastric digestion, prepares the partially digested mixture, known as chyme, for the next stage.

The Small Intestine: The Stage for Nutrient Absorption

Chyme slowly enters the small intestine, a long, convoluted tube divided into the duodenum, jejunum, and ileum. The symphony reaches its crescendo as many digestive enzymes and secretions from the pancreas, liver, and gallbladder converge. Pancreatic enzymes like trypsin, chymotrypsin, and amylase continue the breakdown of proteins, carbohydrates, and fats. Bile, produced by the liver and stored in the gallbladder, emulsifies fats, increasing their surface area for enzymatic action and absorption. The intestinal epithelium, lined with microvilli, provides a vast surface area for nutrient absorption. Specific transporters embedded in the epithelial cells facilitate the uptake of glucose, amino acids, fatty acids, vitamins, and minerals into the bloodstream, marking the culmination of nutrient absorption.

The Grand Finale: Waste Elimination and Gut Microbiome Harmony

Undigested residues and indigestible materials move into the large intestine, also known as the colon. The colon's primary function is water absorption, solidifying the remaining waste into feces. The gut microbiome, a diverse community of trillions of bacteria residing in the colon, plays a crucial role in this final stage.

These microbial residents ferment indigestible carbohydrates, producing short-chain fatty acids (SCFAs) like butyrate, propionate, and acetate. SCFAs nourish the colonic epithelium, contribute to immune function, and regulate various metabolic processes. Finally, the remaining waste is eliminated through the rectum and anus, concluding the digestive symphony.

The Importance of a Healthy Digestive Symphony

Optimal digestive function is integral to overall health and well-being. Efficient nutrient absorption fuels the body's energy needs, supports growth and repair, and bolsters the immune system. Conversely, imbalances or disruptions in the digestive symphony can lead to many health concerns, including nutrient deficiencies, gastrointestinal disorders, and chronic diseases. Maintaining a healthy gut through balanced dietary choices, adequate hydration, stress management, and regular physical activity can ensure the smooth performance of this vital internal orchestra.

References:

- Hall, J. E. (2016). Guyton and Hall textbook of medical physiology (13th ed.). Elsevier.

- Quigley, E. M. A., & Buchman, A. L. (2019). The role of the gut microbiome in nutrition and health. Clinical reviews in food science and nutrition, 59(8), 1449-1499.

- National Institutes of Health. (2021, April 28). Your digestive system & how it works. National Institutes of Health. Retrieved from https://www.niddk.nih.gov/health-information/digestive diseases/digestive-system-how-it-works

Lorenzi R.Marcos

N8: THE DIGESTIVE SYSTEM: CONDUCTING THE ORCHESTRA OF YOUR HEALTH

The digestive system, often seen as a solitary actor, plays a vital role in a grander production—your overall health. Far from operating in isolation, it is the conductor, harmonizing with and influencing the ten other human systems in a complex and essential symphony.

The Immune System: A healthy gut, nurtured by a balanced microbiome, plays a crucial role in immune function. Gut bacteria produce compounds that strengthen the intestinal barrier and modulate immune responses, protecting us from pathogens and inflammation.

The Endocrine System: Hormones produced by the pancreas and gut hormones released by the digestive system work in tandem to regulate blood sugar levels, energy metabolism, and appetite. This intricate dance ensures optimal energy homeostasis.

The Excretory System: The digestive and excretory systems work together to eliminate waste products. The colon absorbs water and forms stool, while the kidneys filter and excrete metabolic waste through urine. Together, they maintain the body's fluid balance and remove harmful substances.

The Integumentary System: The gut microbiome influences the health of the skin, our largest organ. Gut bacteria produce metabolites that can impact skin conditions like eczema and psoriasis, highlighting the interconnectedness of these systems.

The Musculoskeletal System: The nutrients absorbed from food fuel muscle growth and repair, which are essential for movement and maintaining bone health. Physical activity improves gut motility and microbiome diversity, creating a feedback loop.

The Nervous System: The gut and brain constantly communicate through the "gut-brain axis." The enteric nervous system, embedded within the gut, influences mood, stress response, and cognitive function. Conversely, stress can negatively impact gut motility and digestion.

The Reproductive System: Gut health can influence hormone production and fertility in both men and women. The gut microbiome also plays a role in fetal development, highlighting the intergenerational impact of digestive health.

The Respiratory System: While seemingly unrelated, gut inflammation can trigger respiratory issues like asthma and allergies. Maintaining a healthy gut microbiome can offer protection against these conditions.

The Lymphatic System: This network of vessels and tissues is crucial in immune function and waste removal. The lymphatic system works with the digestive system to transport immune cells and absorb dietary fats, demonstrating their integrated functionality.

In conclusion, the digestive system is far from an isolated performer. It conducts a complex and essential symphony, harmonizing with every other system in the body to maintain optimal health. By nurturing a healthy digestive system, we invest in the well-being of our entire being, ensuring a harmonious performance for a vibrant and healthy life.

N9: Food as Information: Decoding the Messages Your Body Reads with Every Bite

Imagine food not just as sustenance but as a language your body understands at its very core. Every morsel you consume carries coded messages that instruct your cells, influence your hormones, and shape your overall health. Understanding this "food as information" concept empowers you to make conscious choices for optimal well-being.

Processed vs. Whole: A Tale of Two Messages Think of processed foods as garbled transmissions with artificial additives, refined sugars, and unhealthy fats. These can confuse your cellular communication, leading to:

- Inflammation

- Blood sugar spikes
- Nutrient deprivation

On the other hand, whole, unprocessed foods act like clear, concise messages. They deliver:

- Essential nutrients
- Balanced energy
- Antioxidant power

Examples of "Speaking" the Cellular Language:

- Leafy greens
- Berries
- Nuts and seeds
- Omega-3 fatty acids
- Colorful vegetables

Mindful Eating: Cultivating a Fluent Dialogue with Food
Engage in mindful eating practices to better understand the messages your body receives:

- Savor each bite
- Listen to your body
- Connect with your food
- Respect your body

By viewing food as information, you can decode the messages your body receives with every bite, making informed choices that support optimal health and vitality. Embrace the language of whole, unprocessed foods, and cultivate a harmonious dialogue between your plate and your cells. Your body will thank you with abundant energy, resilience, and well-being.

CHAPTER 29

N10: THE POWER OF FOOD MEMORIES: HOW TASTE TRIGGERS TIME TRAVEL

Close your eyes and take a bite of your favorite childhood dish. In that moment, you're not just tasting food; you're experiencing a flood of memories, emotions, and sensations. This is the magic of food memories – they transcend taste, triggering a journey through time and space.

The Science Behind Food Memories

Food memories are deeply ingrained in our brains, intertwining with our senses, emotions, and experiences. When we taste familiar flavors, our brains light up with activity, activating memory, emotion, and reward regions. This phenomenon is linked to the hippocampus and amygdala, responsible for memory formation and emotional processing.

Why are food memories so potent?

1. Emotional resonance: Food memories are often tied to significant emotional events, like family gatherings, celebrations, or moments of comfort. The emotional context enhances their impact and longevity.

2. Multi-sensory experience: Food engages multiple senses – taste, smell, sight, touch, and even sound. This rich sensory input creates vivid, multi-dimensional memories that linger in our minds.

3. Cultural and social connections: Food is a fundamental part of culture and identity, shaping our sense of belonging and community. Shared meals and culinary traditions reinforce social bonds and create lasting memories.

4. Neurological wiring: The brain's neural pathways link taste and smell with memory and emotion, creating associative solid connections. This wiring makes food a powerful mnemonic device, remarkably clarifying specific memories.

Harnessing the Power of Food Memories

1. Create new traditions: Incorporate meaningful food rituals into your life, whether a weekly family dinner or a special holiday feast. These shared experiences will become cherished memories for years to come.

2. Explore culinary heritage: Revisit the flavors of your heritage, exploring traditional recipes passed down through generations. Cooking and sharing these dishes can strengthen cultural connections and foster a sense of identity.

3. Document your culinary adventures: Keep a food journal or create a digital photo album documenting your culinary explorations. Capture the dishes and the stories, people, and places behind them.

4. Share meals with loved ones: Break bread with family and friends, sharing laughter, stories, and good food. The act of sharing a meal creates lasting memories and strengthens relationships.

Food memories can transport us across time and space, whether the aroma of freshly baked bread or the taste of a beloved family recipe. Embrace the magic of taste-induced time travel, savoring each moment and cherishing the memories that food brings to life. After all, the most memorable journeys nourish not just the body but also the soul.

The Mind-Gut Connection: A Symphony of Signals

Our digestive journey begins not in the stomach but in the mind. The mere sight, smell, and anticipation of food trigger a symphony of hormonal responses. Saliva production increases, preparing enzymes to break down carbohydrates. Gastric juices begin to flow, anticipating protein and fat digestion. This intricate communication between the mind and gut, mediated by the vagus nerve, lays the foundation for optimal nutrient absorption.

N11 MINDFUL CHEWING: THE MASTER KEY TO DIGESTION

Mindfulness, the practice of paying focused attention to the present moment without judgment, elevates chewing from autopilot to conscious control. Each mindful chew:

- Increases surface area: By breaking down food into smaller particles, you enhance the accessibility of nutrients to digestive enzymes, optimizing absorption.

- Promotes enzyme activity: Chewing stimulates the production of amylase in saliva, the first step in carbohydrate breakdown, easing the burden on the digestive system.

- Slows down the process: Mindful eating encourages slower, more deliberate chewing, allowing for better mixing of food with saliva and digestive enzymes, leading to improved digestion and nutrient uptake.

- Reduces stress: The calming nature of mindful eating counteracts the adverse effects of stress hormones on digestion, promoting a more balanced internal environment.

The Science Speaks: Research supports the power of mindful eating and proper chewing. Studies show that mindful eating practices:

- Increase satiety: Mindful eating can help you eat less and feel more satisfied by promoting awareness of hunger and fullness cues, potentially aiding in weight management.

- Improve digestion: Studies suggest that mindful eating can reduce bloating, constipation, and other digestive discomfort.

- Enhance nutrient absorption: Increased chewing may lead to better absorption of certain nutrients, particularly iron and calcium.

Beyond Digestion: A Holistic Transformation Mindful chewing extends beyond the digestive tract, impacting overall well-being. By fostering a conscious connection with your food, you cultivate:

Lorenzi R.Marcos

- Increased enjoyment: Slowing down and savoring each bite allows you to appreciate your food's authentic flavors and textures, enhancing the experience and promoting a positive relationship with food.

- Reduced stress and anxiety: Mindful eating can be a powerful stress management tool, promoting relaxation and emotional well-being.

- Improved mental clarity: By focusing on the present moment, mindful eating can enhance focus and concentration, boosting cognitive performance.

Chewing for Change: "Incorporating mindful eating and proper chewing practices into your daily life is a transformative journey, one delicious bite at a time. Start by:**

- Setting the scene: Create a calm and distraction-free meal environment.

- Tuning in Before you eat, take a few moments to connect with your body and hunger cues.

- Savoring each bite: Chew slowly and deliberately, focusing on the texture, flavor, and aroma of your food.

- Putting down your fork: Pause between bites to allow your body to register fullness cues.

Remember, mindful eating is a practice, not perfection. Be kind to yourself, celebrate small wins, and experience the joy of a conscious relationship with your food. By embracing this shift, you unlock a deeper connection with your body, optimize your health, and embark on a "chewing for change" journey far beyond the plate.

"The first wealth is health." - Ralph Waldo Emerson, American philosopher.

N12: DEBUNKING COMMON NUTRITION MYTHS:

Myth: Carbs are bad for you. Fact: Complex carbohydrates from whole grains, fruits, and vegetables provide essential energy and fiber, crucial for gut health and overall well-being.

Myth: Detox cleanses are necessary to eliminate toxins. Fact: Your body has efficient detoxification systems; restrictive cleanses can deprive you of vital nutrients and disrupt healthy gut bacteria.

Myth: Spot reduction is possible. Fact: You cannot target fat loss to specific areas; focus on healthy eating and exercise for fat reduction.

Myth: Breakfast is the most important meal of the day. Fact: While eating breakfast can be beneficial, finding a sustainable eating pattern that works for you is the most critical factor.

Myth: Eating late at night leads to weight gain. Fact: Weight gain is primarily determined by overall calorie intake and expenditure, not by the timing of your meals.

Remember:

- Embrace evidence-based approaches: Seek guidance from qualified professionals like registered dietitians or licensed nutritionists for personalized advice.

- Focus on whole, unprocessed foods: Prioritize fruits, vegetables, whole grains, lean proteins, and healthy fats for optimal nutrition.

- Develop mindful eating practices: Savor your food, eat slowly, and avoid distractions to cultivate a healthy relationship with food.

- Listen to your body: Learn your hunger and fullness cues to eat intuitively and avoid restrictive diets.

N13 GUT LEAK: THE STEALTHY CULPRIT AND ITS MURKY SYMPTOMS

While "gut leak" has gained popularity, its scientific basis and symptoms remain multifaceted and open to discussion. Here's a brief overview:

What is a gut leak? "Gut leak" isn't an officially recognized medical term but a hypothesis suggesting increased intestinal permeability. This means the tight junctions between gut cells become compromised, allowing larger molecules like toxins and undigested food particles to leak into the bloodstream.

Symptoms: Symptoms associated with gut leak are often vague and non-specific, making diagnosis challenging. They can include:

- Digestive issues: Bloating, constipation, diarrhea, gas

- Skin problems: Eczema, rosacea, acne

- Fatigue and brain fog

- Autoimmune flares (in individuals with pre-existing conditions)

However, these symptoms do not exclusively point to gut leaks and could be linked to other digestive and systemic conditions.

Key Scientific Studies:

1. **Increased Intestinal Permeability in Patients with Celiac Disease:** This study observed higher intestinal permeability in celiac disease patients compared to healthy individuals, highlighting the association with specific conditions.

2. **Tight Junction Alterations and Intestinal Mucosal Barrier Dysfunction in Moderate to Severe Ulcerative Colitis:** This study identified tight junction disruption in ulcerative colitis patients, suggesting gut leak might be involved in disease progression.

3. **Intestinal Permeability and Its Relevance to Disease:** This review discusses the potential role of

increased intestinal permeability in various diseases, highlighting the complex interplay with other factors.

Important Note: While the research shows promising avenues, evidence directly linking general "gut leak" to specific symptoms and diseases remains limited. More research is needed to establish its validity and potential diagnostic methods. If you experience concerning symptoms, it's crucial to consult a healthcare professional for an accurate diagnosis and appropriate treatment plans. Self-diagnosing and resorting to unproven interventions based on "gut leak" claims can be risky.

Scientific Treatment for Gut Leak: A Nuance-Filled Landscape

While the concept of "gut leak" has gained traction, its treatment remains complex and often contentious. The lack of a definitive diagnostic test and limited large-scale research create challenges in establishing standardized treatment protocols. Here's a breakdown of the current landscape:

Proposed Treatments:

- **Dietary Interventions:** These focus on gut-healing diets, typically emphasizing whole, unprocessed foods, increased fiber intake, and reduced inflammatory triggers like gluten or dairy. While some proponents tout their benefits, studies haven't consistently supported their efficacy across all individuals.

- **Probiotics and Prebiotics:** These supplements restore gut microbial balance, potentially improving gut integrity. While certain strains have shown promise in limited studies, their efficacy varies, and more research is needed to identify optimal formulations and dosages.

- **Medications:** Treatment typically involves medications targeting inflammation and immune dysregulation in cases of underlying conditions contributing to gut leak, such as inflammatory bowel disease (IBD). However, these treatments address the underlying condition rather than the gut leak.

- **Lifestyle Modifications:** Stress management techniques, regular exercise, and adequate sleep are often recommended to support overall gut health. While these lifestyle factors can influence gut function indirectly, their direct impact on gut leak remains unclear.

The Role of Individual Variability: One size does not fit all in gut health treatment. Genetics, microbiome composition, dietary habits, and environmental exposures contribute to individual variability in gut function and response to treatment. Personalized approaches, guided by healthcare professionals, are crucial to address specific needs and optimize outcomes.

Navigating the Nuances: Given the complexity of gut health and the lack of definitive diagnostic markers for gut leaks, navigating treatment options can be challenging. Here are some key considerations:

- **Consult a Healthcare Professional:** Seek guidance from a qualified healthcare provider, such as a gastroenterologist or registered dietitian, for accurate diagnosis and personalized treatment recommendations.

- **Focus on Whole-Person Health:** Addressing gut health involves a holistic approach that considers factors beyond diet and supplements, including stress management, sleep quality, and physical activity.

- **Beware of Quick Fixes:** Be cautious of unproven treatments or products claiming to "cure" gut leaks. Sustainable improvements in gut health often require patience, consistency, and evidence-based interventions.

- **Stay Informed:** Stay updated on emerging research and evidence-based practices in gut health management. Reliable sources such as peer-reviewed journals and reputable healthcare organizations can provide valuable insights.

By navigating the nuances of gut health treatment with informed guidance and a personalized approach, individuals can take proactive steps toward optimizing their digestive well-being and overall health.

CHAPTER 30
N14 MINDFUL MOVEMENT: THE DANCE OF DIGESTION

Just as mindful eating fosters a deeper connection with food, mindful movement cultivates awareness of how physical activity influences digestion. Whether it's yoga, tai chi, or a stroll, incorporating mindful movement into your routine can enhance digestive function and overall well-being.

The Gut-Brain-Movement Connection: The gut-brain axis extends beyond digestion to encompass the intricate interplay between physical activity and mental health. Mindful movement activates the parasympathetic nervous system, promoting relaxation and reducing stress—a critical factor in digestive health. As you move mindfully, you:

- Enhance blood flow: Physical activity increases blood circulation to the digestive organs, facilitating nutrient absorption and waste removal.

- Stimulate peristalsis: Gentle movements massage the intestines, promoting rhythmic contractions that aid digestion and alleviate constipation.

- Alleviate stress: Mindful movement techniques, such as deep breathing and gentle stretching, activate the body's relaxation response, reducing stress hormones that can impair digestion.

- Improve mood: Regular physical activity releases endorphins, neurotransmitters that enhance mood and reduce feelings of anxiety and depression. This fosters a positive mindset conducive to healthy digestion.

Mindful Movement Practices for Digestive Health:

1. **Yoga:** Incorporate yoga poses that target digestion, such as seated twists, gentle forward bends, and abdominal breathing techniques like diaphragmatic breathing (pranayama).

Lorenzi R.Marcos

2. **Tai Chi:** Embrace the slow, flowing movements of tai chi to promote relaxation, balance, and harmony within the body, which can benefit digestive function.

3. **Walking:** Take mindful walks in nature, focusing on each step and breath, to stimulate digestion, reduce stress, and enhance overall well-being.

4. **Qigong:** Engage in qigong exercises that combine gentle movements, breathwork, and meditation to balance the body's energy (qi) and support digestive health.

The Science of Mindful Movement: Research supports the therapeutic benefits of mindful movement for digestive health:

- **Yoga for Irritable Bowel Syndrome (IBS):** Studies suggest that yoga interventions can improve symptoms and quality of life in individuals with IBS by reducing stress and modulating gut function.

- **Tai Chi for Functional Dyspepsia:** Research indicates that tai chi practice may alleviate symptoms of functional dyspepsia, a common digestive disorder, by promoting relaxation and reducing visceral hypersensitivity.

- **Walking for Constipation:** Walking has been shown to stimulate bowel motility and alleviate constipation by increasing abdominal muscle activity and promoting peristalsis.

Embark on a Journey of Mindful Movement: Integrating mindful movement into daily life doesn't require elaborate routines or extensive training. Start with small, achievable steps:

- Begin with gentle activities that resonate with your body and preferences.

- Practice mindful breathing during movement to enhance relaxation and focus.

- Prioritize consistency over intensity, aiming for regular, sustainable practice.

- Listen to your body and honor its cues, adjusting your practice as needed.

As you embark on this mindful movement journey, savor each moment of connection between body, mind, and spirit. By nurturing your body with gentle, intentional movement, you foster a harmonious relationship with your digestive system, promoting optimal health and vitality.

N15 THE JOURNEY OF MINDFUL DIGESTION: CULTIVATING AWARENESS FROM PLATE TO STOMACH

Embark on a journey of mindful digestion, where each bite becomes a sacred act of nourishment and connection. By cultivating awareness from plate to stomach, you unlock the transformative power of mindful eating, fostering optimal digestion and overall well-being.

The Art of Mindful Eating: Mindful eating is more than just a technique; it's a way of life that invites you to engage all your senses and honor the food journey from farm to fork. Here's how to embrace mindful eating:

1. Pause and Reflect: Before you eat, take a moment to pause and connect with your body. Notice any sensations of hunger or fullness and any emotions or thoughts present in the moment.

2. Engage Your Senses: As you prepare your meal, engage your senses fully. Notice the colors, textures, and aromas of the food before you. Take pleasure in the act of cooking and savoring each ingredient.

3. Chew Slowly and Thoroughly: Mindful chewing begins with taking smaller bites and chewing each morsel slowly and thoroughly. Please pay attention to the taste and texture of the food as it transforms in your mouth.

4. Tune into Your Body: Check in with your body periodically throughout the meal. Notice any hunger or fullness signals changes, and honor them by eating according to your body's needs.

5. Cultivate Gratitude: Practice gratitude for the food on your plate and the nourishment it provides. Reflect on the journey of each ingredient and the hands that brought it to you.

The Science of Mindful Digestion: Research demonstrates the profound impact of mindful eating on digestion and overall health:

- Reduced Stress Response: Mindful eating reduces cortisol levels and activates the parasympathetic nervous system, promoting relaxation and optimal digestive function.

- Enhanced Nutrient Absorption: Slowing down the eating process and thoroughly chewing food optimizes the breakdown of nutrients and facilitates absorption in the digestive tract.

- Improved Gut-Brain Communication: Mindful eating enhances communication between the brain and gut, leading to better digestion, nutrient uptake, and overall gut health.

Embrace the Journey of Mindful Digestion: As you embark on mindful digestion, remember that it's not about perfection but progress. Here are some tips to guide you along the way:

- Start Small: Begin by incorporating mindful eating practices into one meal each day. Gradually expand your mindfulness to other meals and snacks as you become more comfortable.

- Practice Patience: Mindful digestion is a skill that takes time to develop. Be patient with yourself and embrace the process, knowing that each mindful bite brings you closer to optimal health.

- Seek Support: Connect with like-minded individuals who share your journey toward mindful eating. Joining a community or finding a mindfulness partner can provide encouragement and accountability.

- Celebrate Successes: Celebrate your victories, no matter how small. Whether choosing a nourishing meal or savoring a mindful bite, each step forward is worth acknowledging and celebrating.

You nourish your body, mind, and spirit by embracing mindful digestion. With each mindful bite, you cultivate a deeper connection with yourself and the world, fostering health, harmony, and wholeness.

N16 UNDERSTANDING THE GUT-BRAIN CONNECTION: UNRAVELING THE MYSTERIES OF DIGESTIVE HEALTH

The gut-brain connection is a complex and intricate network fundamental to digestive health and overall well-being. From mood regulation to immune function, this dynamic relationship between the gut and the brain influences virtually every aspect of human physiology. Let's explore the science behind the gut-brain connection and its implications for digestive health.

The Gut-Brain Axis: The gut-brain axis is a bidirectional communication pathway that links the central nervous system (CNS) with the gastrointestinal tract's enteric nervous system (ENS). This two-way communication occurs via neural, hormonal, and immunological signaling pathways, facilitating constant interaction between the gut and the brain.

Critical Components of the Gut-Brain Axis:

1. Enteric Nervous System (ENS): Often referred to as the "second brain," the ENS consists of a complex network of neurons that governs gastrointestinal motility, secretion, and absorption. It operates autonomously and communicates via the vagus nerve with the central nervous system.

2. Vagus Nerve: The vagus nerve is a significant conduit for bidirectional communication between the gut and the brain. It transmits sensory information from the gut to the brain and carries motor signals from the brain to the stomach, regulating various digestive processes.

3. Neurotransmitters: The gut produces many neurotransmitters, including serotonin, dopamine, and gamma-aminobutyric acid (GABA), crucial in mood regulation, appetite control, and gastrointestinal function.

4. Gut Microbiota: The gut microbiota, composed of trillions of bacteria, fungi, and other microorganisms, influences gut-brain communication by producing neurotransmitters, short-chain fatty acids (SCFAs), and other bioactive compounds.

Implications for Digestive Health: The gut-brain connection profoundly affects digestive health. It impacts conditions such as irritable bowel syndrome (IBS), inflammatory bowel disease (IBD), and functional dyspepsia. Dysregulation of the gut-brain axis can lead to gastrointestinal symptoms, including abdominal pain, bloating, diarrhea, and constipation.

Furthermore, emerging research suggests that disturbances in gut-brain communication may contribute to the pathogenesis of psychiatric disorders such as depression, anxiety, and autism spectrum disorders. This highlights the interconnectedness of mental and digestive health and underscores the importance of addressing both aspects in clinical practice.

Therapeutic Approaches: Understanding the gut-brain connection opens new avenues for therapeutic intervention in treating digestive disorders and mental health conditions.

Promising approaches include:

- Probiotics and Prebiotics: Modulating the gut microbiota with probiotics and prebiotics may help restore balance to the gut-brain axis, alleviating symptoms of digestive disorders and improving mood and cognition.

- Dietary Interventions: Certain dietary patterns, such as the Mediterranean and low-FODMAP diets, have been shown to positively influence gut-brain communication and reduce symptoms of IBS and IBD.

- Mind-Body Therapies: Mindfulness-based interventions, cognitive-behavioral therapy (CBT), and gut-directed hypnotherapy can help regulate the stress response and enhance gut-brain communication, improving digestive health and mental well-being.

By unraveling the mysteries of the gut-brain connection, researchers shed light on the profound interplay between the gut and the brain. As our understanding deepens, so will our ability to develop innovative therapies that promote optimal digestive health and holistic well-being.

Lorenzi R.Marcos

CHAPTER 31

N17 MINDFUL EATING: NOURISHING BODY, MIND, AND SPIRIT

Mindful eating is a transformative practice that invites us to cultivate awareness, intention, and gratitude in our relationship with food. We nourish our bodies, minds, and spirits by savoring each bite with presence and reverence, fostering holistic well-being and a deeper connection to the world.

The Essence of Mindful Eating:

At its core, mindful eating brings mindfulness—moment-to-moment awareness—to the eating experience. It involves tuning into our body's hunger and fullness cues, savoring the flavors and textures of food, and cultivating gratitude for the nourishment it provides.

Critical Principles of Mindful Eating:

1. **Presence:** Mindful eating begins with bringing full awareness to the present moment. By slowing down and tuning into our senses, we can fully experience eating without distractions.

2. **Non-Judgment:** Mindful eating encourages us to observe our thoughts and emotions without judgment. Instead of labeling foods as "good" or "bad," we approach eating with curiosity and self-compassion.

3. **Gratitude:** Cultivating gratitude for the food on our plate and the hands that prepared it enhances our appreciation for the nourishment it provides. We acknowledge the interconnectedness of all beings involved in the food chain.

4. **Intuition:** Trusting our body's innate wisdom, we honor its hunger and fullness cues and make food choices that align with our physical and emotional needs. We eat for nourishment and pleasure rather than out of habit or external rules.

5. **Mindful Awareness:** By paying attention to the sensations of hunger, fullness, and satisfaction, we develop a deeper

understanding of our body's needs and preferences. We become attuned to the subtle signals guiding us in conscious choices about what, when, and how much to eat.

Benefits of Mindful Eating:

The practice of mindful eating offers a myriad of benefits for body, mind, and spirit:

- **Improved Digestion:** By slowing down and chewing food thoroughly, we aid digestion and enhance nutrient absorption, reducing symptoms of indigestion and bloating.

- **Enhanced Awareness:** Mindful eating heightens our sensory awareness, allowing us to fully appreciate the flavors, textures, and aromas of food. We develop a deeper connection to the culinary experience.

- **Weight Management:** By eating mindfully and tuning into our body's hunger and fullness cues, we become more attuned to our natural appetite and are less likely to overeat or indulge in emotional eating.

- **Reduced Stress:** Mindful eating promotes relaxation and reduces stress by activating the body's parasympathetic nervous system. We approach meals with a sense of calm and ease, free from the distractions of the mind.

- **Greater Satisfaction:** We derive greater satisfaction from our meals by savoring each bite and eating with intention. We feel more nourished, fulfilled, and content, both physically and emotionally.

Practical Tips for Mindful Eating:

Incorporate the following practices into your daily routine to cultivate mindful eating:

- **Eat Without Distractions:** Avoid distractions like television, smartphones, or computers while eating. Instead, focus solely on eating and the sensory experience it provides.

- **Slow Down:** Take your time chewing each bite thoroughly and savoring the flavors of the food. Put your utensils between bites and pause to listen to your body's hunger and fullness signals.

- **Practice Gratitude:** Before each meal, take a moment to express gratitude for the food on your plate and the nourishment it provides. Reflect on the journey of each ingredient and the hands that brought it to you.

- **Listen to Your Body:** Tune into your body's hunger and fullness cues, eating when you're hungry and stopping when you're satisfied. Honor your body's wisdom and trust its innate ability to guide you in nourishing choices.

- **Be Curious:** Approach eating with curiosity and an open mind. Explore new foods and flavors with a sense of wonder and experimentation. Notice how different foods affect your body and mood.

By embracing mindful eating, we can transform our relationship with food from mindless consumption to conscious nourishment. Each mindful bite cultivates a deeper connection to ourselves, food, and the world, fostering health, happiness, and wholeness.

N18 THE POWER OF MINDFUL MOVEMENT: INTEGRATING BODY, BREATH, AND MIND

Mindful movement is a practice that invites us to cultivate awareness, presence, and connection through intentional movement and conscious breathing. By integrating body, breath, and mind, we tap into the transformative power of movement as a vehicle for self-discovery, healing, and inner peace.

The Essence of Mindful Movement: At its core, mindful movement brings non-judgmental awareness to the experience of moving our bodies. Whether through yoga, tai chi, qigong, or other forms of movement, the focus is on fully present in each moment, observing sensations, thoughts, and emotions without attachment or aversion.

Critical Elements of Mindful Movement:

1. **Breath Awareness:** Mindful movement begins with cultivating awareness of the breath. By synchronizing movement with the breath, we anchor ourselves in the present moment and develop a sense of calm and centeredness.

2. **Body Sensations:** As we move our bodies mindfully, we pay attention to the sensations that arise—such as the stretch of muscles, the rhythm of breath, and the feeling of connection to the earth. We observe these sensations with curiosity and openness.

3. **Mindful Attention:** Mindful movement involves directing our attention inward, tuning into the subtle nuances of our experience. We notice thoughts and emotions as they arise, allowing them to come and go without judgment.

4. **Intentional Movement:** Each movement in mindful practice is deliberate and performed with awareness and purpose. Whether it's a yoga pose, a qigong movement, or a simple stretch, we approach it with mindfulness and reverence.

5. **Presence in Motion:** Mindful movement is not about achieving a perfect pose or performance; it's about being

present in the movement process itself. We let go of striving and instead embrace a sense of ease and flow.

Benefits of Mindful Movement: The practice of mindful movement offers a wide range of benefits for physical, mental, and emotional well-being:

- **Improved Flexibility and Strength:** Mindful movement practices such as yoga and tai chi help improve flexibility, strength, and balance, leading to greater physical vitality and resilience.

- **Stress Reduction:** Mindful movement promotes relaxation and reduces stress by activating the body's relaxation response. It helps calm the nervous system and quiet the mind, fostering a sense of inner peace and tranquility.

- **Enhanced Mind-Body Connection:** By integrating body, breath, and mind, mindful movement deepens our awareness of the interconnectedness of our physical, mental, and emotional experiences. We cultivate a greater sense of wholeness and integration.

- **Emotional Regulation:** Mindful movement provides a safe space to explore and process emotions through movement. It allows us to release tension and energy stored in the body, promoting emotional balance and well-being.

- **Increased Mindfulness:** Regular mindful movement practice strengthens our daily mindfulness capacity. We learn to bring awareness and presence to all activities, fostering a more profound sense of connection and meaning.

Practical Tips for Mindful Movement: Incorporate the following practices into your daily routine to cultivate mindful movement:

- **Choose Activities Mindfully:** Select movement practices that resonate with you and bring you joy, whether it's yoga, tai chi, dance, or walking in nature. Listen to your body and honor its needs and preferences.

- **Start Slowly:** Begin with gentle, accessible movements and gradually increase intensity as you build strength and flexibility. Pay attention to your body's feedback and adjust the intensity as needed.

- **Focus on the Breath:** Use the breath as a guide for movement, coordinating each movement with the inhalation and exhalation. Notice how the breath influences the quality of movement and vice versa.

- **Practice Non-Judgment:** Approach mindful movement with curiosity and self-compassion. Let go of expectations and perfectionism and instead embrace the process of exploration and self-discovery.

- **Cultivate Gratitude:** Express gratitude for your body's ability to move and for the opportunity to engage in mindful movement. Acknowledge the interconnectedness of body, breath, and mind, and honor the sacredness of the present moment.

By embracing mindful movement, we embark on self-discovery and transformation. With each conscious breath and intentional movement, we deepen our connection to ourselves and the world, nurturing holistic well-being and inner peace.

N19 THE HEALING POWER OF NATURE: RECONNECTING WITH THE NATURAL WORLD FOR OPTIMAL HEALTH

Nature has long been revered for its healing properties, offering solace, rejuvenation, and restoration to body, mind, and spirit. In today's fast-paced world, reconnecting with nature is more important than ever as we seek refuge from the stresses of modern life and strive to cultivate optimal health and well-being.

The Healing Essence of Nature: Nature holds a unique power to heal and nurture us on multiple levels:

- **Physical Healing:** Spending time in nature has been shown to reduce blood pressure, lower stress hormones, and boost the immune system. The natural world's sights, sounds, and smells calm the nervous system, promoting relaxation and overall health.

- **Mental and Emotional Well-Being:** Nature has a profound impact on mental and emotional well-being, reducing symptoms of anxiety, depression, and mood disorders. The beauty and tranquility of natural landscapes evoke feelings of awe, wonder, and connection, lifting our spirits and fostering a sense of inner peace.

- **Spiritual Connection:** Nature provides a sacred space for contemplation, reflection, and spiritual renewal. Whether through meditation in the forest, yoga on the beach, or simply sitting beneath a tree, we can connect with something greater than ourselves and tap into a more profound sense of meaning and purpose.

The Science of Nature Therapy: The therapeutic benefits of nature have been widely studied and documented:

- **Forest Bathing:** Forest bathing, or shinrin-yoku, is a Japanese practice that involves immersing oneself in the sights, sounds, and smells of the forest. Research shows that forest bathing reduces stress, lowers blood pressure, and boosts immune function, improving overall health and well-being.

- **Ecotherapy:** Ecotherapy, also known as nature therapy or green therapy, involves engaging in outdoor activities and exercises to promote mental and emotional healing. Whether gardening, hiking, or wildlife observation, ecotherapy offers a holistic approach to wellness that integrates body, mind, and spirit.

- **Biophilia Hypothesis:** The biophilia hypothesis suggests that humans have an innate affinity for nature and that contact with the natural world is essential for psychological and physiological health. Studies have shown that exposure to nature improves mood, enhances cognitive function, and promotes social cohesion.

Practical Tips for Reconnecting with Nature: Incorporate the following practices into your daily life to reap the healing benefits of nature:

- **Spend Time Outdoors:** Make time each day to spend time outdoors, whether it's going for a walk in the park, sitting in your backyard, or taking a hike in the wilderness. Even a few minutes of outdoor time can significantly impact your mood and well-being.

- **Engage Your Senses:** Take time to engage your senses fully and appreciate the natural world's beauty. Notice the colors of the flowers, the scent of the trees, the sound of birdsong, and the feel of the earth beneath your feet.

- **Practice Mindfulness:** Use nature as a backdrop for mindfulness practice. Bring awareness to the present moment and observe your thoughts and emotions as they arise. Notice how nature reflects the impermanence and interconnectedness of all things.

- **Connect with the Elements:** Take time to connect with the elements of nature—earth, air, water, and fire. Whether grounding yourself barefoot on the planet, breathing in the fresh air, swimming in a lake, or sitting by a campfire, allow yourself to feel a sense of belonging and connection to the natural world.

- **Cultivate a Nature Ritual:** Establish a regular nature ritual that allows you to reconnect with the earth's rhythms and the seasons' cycles. Whether it's a daily sunrise walk, a weekly picnic in the park, or a monthly camping trip, find meaningful ways to incorporate nature into your life.

By reconnecting with the healing power of nature, we can cultivate optimal health and well-being, nurturing our body, mind, and spirit in harmony with the natural world. As we embrace our deep connection to the earth and all living beings, we tap into a source of wisdom, strength, and vitality that sustains us on our journey toward wholeness.

N20 CREATING SACRED SPACE: CULTIVATING TRANQUILITY AND HARMONY IN YOUR ENVIRONMENT

Creating sacred space is a powerful practice that invites us to cultivate tranquility, harmony, and inspiration in our surroundings. Whether it's a physical space in our home, a natural setting outdoors, or an inner sanctuary within our hearts, sacred space is a refuge for rest, reflection, and renewal.

The Essence of Sacred Space: At its core, sacred space is a container for the energy of love, peace, and divine presence. It is a space infused with intention where we can connect with our innermost selves and the sacredness of life itself. Sacred space honors the interconnectedness of all things and invites us to dwell in the beauty and mystery of the present moment.

Critical Elements of Sacred Space:

1. **Intention:** Sacred space begins with intention—the conscious decision to create a space infused with love, beauty, and harmony. Whether it's a meditation altar, a garden sanctuary, or a cozy reading nook, the intention behind the space sets the tone for its energy and ambiance.

2. **Beauty:** Beauty is a fundamental aspect of sacred space, evoking awe, wonder, and reverence. Incorporate elements of beauty such as flowers, artwork, candles, and holy symbols to uplift the spirit and inspire the soul.

3. **Harmony:** Sacred space is characterized by a sense of harmony and balance, both visually and energetically. Arrange furniture, objects, and decor to promote flow and movement, allowing energy to circulate freely throughout the space.

4. **Presence:** Presence is the heart of sacred space, inviting us to be fully present in the moment and attuned to its subtle energies. Cultivate mindfulness and awareness as you enter the space, enveloping yourself in its tranquility and grace.

5. **Connection:** Sacred space facilitates connection to oneself, others, and the divine. Whether through meditation, prayer, or simply being in the presence of loved ones, sacred space provides a container for deepening our connections and relationships.

Benefits of Sacred Space: Creating sacred space offers a multitude of benefits for body, mind, and spirit:

- **Stress Reduction:** Sacred space provides a refuge from the stresses of daily life, allowing us to unwind, relax, and recharge. Spending time in a sacred space promotes relaxation and rejuvenation, reducing symptoms of stress and anxiety.

- **Inner Peace:** Sacred space cultivates a sense of inner peace and tranquility, allowing us to find refuge during chaos and uncertainty. It serves as a sanctuary for stillness and reflection, fostering a deeper connection to our innermost selves.

- **Inspiration and Creativity:** Sacred space inspires creativity and imagination, providing a fertile ground for emerging ideas, insights, and inspiration. Whether writing, painting or simply daydreaming, this sacred space encourages us to tap into our creative potential and express ourselves authentically.

- **Spiritual Growth:** Sacred space supports spiritual growth and development, providing a container for meditation, prayer, and contemplation. It serves as a gateway to the divine, facilitating connection with something greater than ourselves and deepening our understanding of the sacredness of life.

- **Connection to Nature:** Sacred space reconnects us with the natural world, reminding us of our interconnectedness with all living beings. Whether it's a garden sanctuary or a sacred grove in the woods, sacred space allows us to commune with the beauty and wisdom of the earth, fostering a sense of reverence and stewardship.

Practical Tips for Creating Sacred Space: Incorporate the following practices into your life to create sacred space and cultivate tranquility and harmony in your environment:

- **Set an Intention:** Begin by setting an intention for your sacred space—to cultivate peace, inspire creativity, or deepen spiritual connection. Allow your intention to guide your choices as you create the space.

- **Clear and Cleanse:** Clear clutter and energetically cleanse the space to remove any stagnant or negative energy. Use techniques such as smudging with sage or palo santo, ringing bells, or playing soothing music to purify the space and invite positive energy.

- **Choose Meaningful Symbols:** Select symbols and objects that hold personal significance and meaning for you. Choose items that evoke joy, inspiration, and connection, whether crystals, sacred artwork, or spiritual statues.

- **Incorporate Natural Elements:** Bring elements of nature into your sacred space to evoke a sense of harmony and connection. Let nature guide you as you decorate the space, whether fresh flowers, potted plants, or natural materials such as wood and stone.

- **Personalize the Space:** Make it your own by infusing it with your personality, interests, and values. Display photographs, souvenirs, and keepsakes that bring you joy and remind you of what is sacred and meaningful in your life.

- **Cultivate Daily Rituals:** Establish daily rituals and practices that allow you to connect with your sacred space regularly. Whether it's lighting a candle, saying a prayer, or simply sitting in silent meditation, find ways to honor the sacredness of the space and nourish your soul.

- **Share the Space:** Invite others to share in the beauty and blessings of your sacred space, whether it's friends, family, or spiritual community. Sacred space becomes even more powerful when shared and celebrated with others.

By creating sacred space in our lives, we cultivate an environment of tranquility, harmony, and inspiration that supports our well-being and spiritual growth. Whether it's a physical space in our home, a natural setting in the outdoors, or an inner sanctuary within our hearts, sacred space serves as a reminder of the beauty and sacredness of life itself, inviting us to dwell in the presence of love, peace, and divine grace.

CHAPTER 32

THE DIGESTIVE SYMPHONY: AN ORCHESTRATED JOURNEY OF NUTRIENTS FROM MOUTH TO GUT

The human digestive system, a marvel of biological engineering, operates with the intricate coordination of multiple organs and processes. This "digestive symphony" begins when food enters the mouth and culminates in absorbing vital nutrients essential for life. Each stage is crucial in converting complex molecules into bioavailable components, influencing physical health and overall well-being.

The Overture: Mechanical Breakdown and Enzymatic Symphony

The journey commences in the mouth, where food is physically fragmented by teeth and mixed with saliva. Salivary amylase initiates the chemical breakdown of carbohydrates, while other enzymes begin the digestion of proteins and fats. This orchestrated process, termed oral digestion, prepares the bolus for swallowing and further breakdown in the stomach.

The Esophageal Interlude: A Muscular Passage

Following chewing and swallowing, the bolus embarks on a brief but essential journey through the esophagus, a muscular tube lined with epithelial tissue. Rhythmic contractions, known as peristalsis, propel the food mass downward, aided by gravity. Sphincters at both ends of the esophagus ensure unidirectional flow, preventing reflux and protecting respiratory pathways.

The Stomach: A Powerful Mixing Vessel and Chemical Cauldron

The stomach, a muscular sac-like organ, serves as the central processing unit of the digestive system. Powerful muscular contractions churn and mix the bolus with gastric juices, a potent cocktail of gastric acid, enzymes, and mucus. Gastric acid, with its low pH, denatures proteins and activates pepsin, an enzyme that further breaks down protein chains. The churning action facilitates the physical breakdown of food particles, increasing their surface area for enzymatic action. This phase, termed gastric digestion, prepares the partially digested mixture, known as chyme, for the next stage.

The Small Intestine: The Stage for Nutrient Absorption

Chyme slowly enters the small intestine, a long, convoluted tube divided into the duodenum, jejunum, and ileum. The symphony reaches its crescendo as many digestive enzymes and secretions from the pancreas, liver, and gallbladder converge. Pancreatic enzymes like trypsin, chymotrypsin, and amylase continue the breakdown of proteins, carbohydrates, and fats. Bile, produced by the liver and stored in the gallbladder, emulsifies fats, increasing their surface area for enzymatic action and absorption. The intestinal epithelium, lined with microvilli, provides a vast surface area for nutrient absorption. Specific transporters embedded in the epithelial cells facilitate the uptake of glucose, amino acids, fatty acids, vitamins, and minerals into the bloodstream, marking the culmination of nutrient absorption.

The Grand Finale: Waste Elimination and Gut Microbiome Harmony

Undigested residues and indigestible materials move into the large intestine, also known as the colon. The colon's primary function is water absorption, solidifying the remaining waste into feces. The gut microbiome, a diverse community of trillions of bacteria residing in the colon, plays a crucial role in this final stage. These microbial residents ferment indigestible carbohydrates, producing short-chain fatty acids (SCFAs) like butyrate, propionate, and acetate. SCFAs nourish the colonic epithelium, contribute to immune function, and regulate various metabolic processes. Finally, the remaining waste is eliminated through the rectum and anus, concluding the digestive symphony.

The Importance of a Healthy Digestive Symphony

Optimal digestive function is integral to overall health and well-being. Efficient nutrient absorption fuels the body's energy needs, supports growth and repair, and bolsters the immune system. Conversely, imbalances or disruptions in the digestive symphony can lead to many health concerns, including nutrient deficiencies, gastrointestinal disorders, and chronic diseases. Maintaining a healthy gut through balanced dietary choices, adequate hydration, stress management, and regular physical activity can ensure the smooth performance of this vital internal orchestra.

References:

- Hall, J. E. (2016). Guyton and Hall textbook of medical physiology (13th ed.). Elsevier.

- Quigley, E. M. A., & Buchman, A. L. (2019). The role of the gut microbiome in nutrition and health. Clinical reviews in food science and nutrition, 59(8), 1449-1499.

- National Institutes of Health. (2021, April 28). Your digestive system & how it works. National Institutes of Health. Retrieved from https://www.niddk.nih.gov/health-information/digestive-diseases/digestive-system-how-it-works

THE DIGESTIVE SYSTEM: CONDUCTING THE ORCHESTRA OF YOUR HEALTH

The digestive system, often seen as a solitary actor, plays a vital role in a grander production—your overall health. Far from operating in isolation, it is the conductor, harmonizing with and influencing the ten other human systems in a complex and essential symphony.

The Circulatory System: The digested nutrients, broken down into elementary forms, enter the bloodstream through the circulatory system. This vital highway delivers the building blocks for energy, growth, and repair to every corner of the body.

The Immune System: A healthy gut, nurtured by a balanced microbiome, plays a crucial role in immune function. Gut bacteria produce compounds that strengthen the intestinal barrier and modulate immune responses, protecting us from pathogens and inflammation.

The Endocrine System: Hormones produced by the pancreas and gut hormones released by the digestive system work in tandem to regulate blood sugar levels, energy metabolism, and appetite. This intricate dance ensures optimal energy homeostasis.

The Excretory System: The digestive and excretory systems work together to eliminate waste products. The colon absorbs water and forms stool, while the kidneys filter and excrete metabolic waste through urine. Together, they maintain the body's fluid balance and remove harmful substances.

The Integumentary System: The gut microbiome influences the health of the skin, our largest organ. Gut bacteria produce metabolites that can impact skin conditions like eczema and psoriasis, highlighting the interconnectedness of these systems.

The Musculoskeletal System: The nutrients absorbed from food fuel muscle growth and repair, which are essential for movement and maintaining bone health. Physical activity improves gut motility and microbiome diversity, creating a feedback loop.

The Nervous System: The gut and brain constantly communicate through the "gut-brain axis." The enteric nervous system, embedded within the gut, influences mood, stress response,

Lorenzi R.Marcos

and cognitive function. Conversely, stress can negatively impact gut motility and digestion.

The Reproductive System: Gut health can influence hormone production and fertility in men and women. The gut microbiome also plays a role in fetal development, highlighting the intergenerational impact of digestive health.

The Respiratory System: While seemingly unrelated, gut inflammation can trigger respiratory issues like asthma and allergies. Maintaining a healthy gut microbiome can offer protection against these conditions.

The Lymphatic System: This network of vessels and tissues is crucial in immune function and waste removal. The lymphatic system works with the digestive system to transport immune cells and absorb dietary fats, demonstrating their integrated functionality.

In conclusion, the digestive system is far from an isolated performer. It conducts a complex and essential symphony, harmonizing with every other system in the body to maintain optimal health. By nurturing a healthy digestive system, we invest in the well-being of our entire being, ensuring a harmonious performance for a vibrant and healthy life.

CHAPTER 33

GROCERY SHOPPING WITH CONFIDENCE: FUELING YOUR BODY FOR OPTIMAL HEALTH

Before you even step foot in the supermarket, take a deep breath and envision a shopping cart filled with vibrant colors, diverse textures, and the building blocks of a Healthy You! Ditch the impulse buys and aim for conscious, informed choices that fuel your body and mind! But first, let's clear the nutritional fog!

UNDERSTANDING YOUR FUEL GAUGE: MACRONUTRIENTS VS. MICRONUTRIENTS

Imagine your body as a high-performance car! To run smoothly, it needs the right fuel in the proper proportions. Here's the breakdown:

- **Macronutrients**: These provide the bulk of your energy and include:

    - **Carbohydrates**: Carbohydrates are your body's readily available energy source, and they are found in fruits, vegetables, grains, and legumes. Choose complex carbs for sustained energy and fiber!

    - **Proteins**: Essential for building and repairing tissues, found in meat, fish, eggs, dairy, legumes, and nuts. Aim for a variety of protein sources to ensure complete amino acid profiles!

    - **Fats**: Don't demonize them! Healthy fats are crucial for brain function, hormone production, and nutrient absorption. Opt for unsaturated fats from avocado, olive oil, nuts, and fatty fish!

- **Micronutrients**: These are the essential vitamins and minerals your body needs in smaller amounts for various functions:

    - **Vitamins**: Supporting immunity, metabolism, and organ function (found in diverse fruits, vegetables, and fortified foods).

    - **Minerals**: Crucial for bone health, enzyme function, and nerve impulse transmission (found in fruits, vegetables, nuts, seeds, and dairy).

CHOOSING YOUR DIETARY PATH: EXPLORING OPTIONS WITH CONFIDENCE

With basic nutrition knowledge, you can approach different dietary approaches with an informed lens. Here are some popular options:

- **Balanced Diet**: This flexible approach emphasizes variety and moderation from all food groups, prioritizing whole foods and limiting processed options.

  - *Pros*: Sustainable, nutrient-rich, and adaptable to individual needs.

  - *Cons*: Requires planning and awareness.

- **Vegetarian**: Excludes meat and poultry, focusing on plant-based proteins like legumes, nuts, and eggs.

  - *Pros*: Rich in fiber, potentially lowers the risk of certain chronic diseases.

  - *Cons*: Requires careful planning to ensure adequate protein and certain nutrients.

- **Vegan**: Excludes all animal products, including meat, dairy, and eggs.

  - *Pros*: Promotes animal welfare and may offer environmental benefits.

  - *Cons*: Demands meticulous planning to ensure nutrient sufficiency.

Resources for Informed Choices

- **Vegan Society**: Founded in 1944, the Vegan Society is the world's oldest vegan organization, headquartered in the UK. They offer information, resources, and support for individuals and businesses transitioning to a vegan lifestyle.

- **Vegetarian Resource Group (VRG)**: Established in 1985, the VRG is a leading North American organization that provides information and resources on vegetarian and vegan diets. They offer extensive nutritional guidance, recipes, and advocacy resources.

- **The Humane Society of the United States (HSUS)**: Founded in 1877, the HSUS is a large non-profit organization that advocates for animal welfare and promotes plant-based diets to reduce animal cruelty and environmental impact.

- **MyPlate**: The United States Department of Agriculture (USDA) provides a visual guide to balanced, healthy eating. It divides a plate into five sections representing different food groups: fruits, vegetables, grains, protein foods, and dairy. This resource provides simple, easy-to-understand guidance on creating balanced meals with the right proportions of different food groups.

International References

- **World Health Organization (WHO)**: WHO provides various resources on healthy eating, including information on specific nutrients, dietary advice for different populations, and global nutrition issues.

- **Food and Agriculture Organization of the United Nations (FAO)**: FAO resources explore sustainable food systems, food security, and healthy diets. They offer guidelines and tools for different stakeholder groups.

- **Global Food Safety Partnership (GFSP)**: GFSP focuses on food safety and provides resources and tools for consumers, industry, and governments to ensure safe food practices. It raises awareness about food safety concerns and empowers informed choices regarding food selection and handling.

- **International Food Safety Authorities Network (INFOSAN)**: INFOSAN facilitates rapid international response to foodborne illness outbreaks and provides crucial information regarding potential food safety risks for consumers and authorities.

FOOD AS INFORMATION: DECODING THE MESSAGES YOUR BODY READS WITH EVERY BITE

Imagine food as sustenance and a language your body understands at its very core! Every morsel you consume carries coded messages that instruct your cells, influence your hormones, and shape your overall health.

Processed vs. Whole: A Tale of Two Messages

Think of processed foods as garbled transmissions with artificial additives, refined sugars, and unhealthy fats! These can confuse your cellular communication, leading to:

- *Inflammation*: The body misinterprets processed messages as threats, triggering chronic inflammation, a cause of numerous diseases.

- *Blood sugar spikes*: Refined sugars send misleading signals, causing insulin surges and crashes, disrupting energy levels, and potentially leading to diabetes.

- *Nutrient deprivation*: Stripped of their natural fiber and essential vitamins, these foods leave your cells starving for optimal information.

On the other hand, whole, unprocessed foods act like clear, concise messages. They deliver:

- *Essential nutrients*: Vitamins, minerals, and phytonutrients provide cells with the building blocks and instructions they need to function optimally.

- *Balanced energy*: Complex carbohydrates release sustained energy, preventing blood sugar fluctuations and promoting focus.

- *Antioxidant power*: Natural antioxidants combat free radical damage, protecting cells and promoting healthy aging.

Examples of "Speaking" the Cellular Language

- *Leafy greens*: Packed with vitamins A, C, and K, they speak of solid immunity, vibrant skin, and healthy bones.

- *Berries*: Bursting with antioxidants, they whisper of reduced inflammation and cellular protection.

- *Fatty fish*: Rich in omega-3 fatty acids, they convey improved cognitive function, heart health, and reduced inflammation.

- *Nuts and seeds*: Delivering protein, fiber, and healthy fats, they signal satiety, sustained energy, and improved cholesterol levels.

The Call to Awareness

You actively participate in your cellular dialogue by choosing whole, unprocessed foods. You empower your body to thrive, combat chronic diseases, and unlock its full potential. Embrace this knowledge, become a mindful eater, and rewrite your health story, one delicious, informative bite at a time!

Remember!

- Prioritize fresh fruits, vegetables, whole grains, lean protein, and healthy fats!

- Limit processed foods, sugary drinks, and unhealthy fats!

- Consult a registered dietitian for personalized guidance!

Let's raise awareness about the power of "food as information" and inspire others to nourish their bodies with the messages they deserve! We can create a healthier, happier world, one informed bite at a time.

CHAPTER 34

GUT LEAK: THE STEALTHY CULPRIT AND ITS MURKY SYMPTOMS

While "gut leak" has gained popularity, its scientific basis and symptoms remain multifaceted and open to discussion. Here's a brief overview:

WHAT IS A GUT LEAK?

"Gut leak" isn't an officially recognized medical term but a hypothesis suggesting increased intestinal permeability. This means the tight junctions between gut cells become compromised, allowing larger molecules like toxins and undigested food particles to leak into the bloodstream.

Symptoms:

Symptoms associated with gut leak are often vague and non-specific, making diagnosis challenging. They can include:

- Digestive issues: Bloating, constipation, diarrhea, gas

- Skin problems: Eczema, rosacea, acne

- Fatigue and brain fog

- Autoimmune flares (in individuals with pre-existing conditions)

However, these symptoms do not exclusively point to gut leaks and could be linked to other digestive and systemic conditions.

Key Scientific Studies:

1. **Increased Intestinal Permeability in Patients with Celiac Disease:** This study observed higher intestinal permeability in celiac disease patients compared to healthy individuals, highlighting the association with specific conditions.

2. **Tight Junction Alterations and Intestinal Mucosal Barrier Dysfunction in Moderate to Severe Ulcerative Colitis:** This study identified tight junction

disruption in ulcerative colitis patients, suggesting gut leak might be involved in disease progression.

3. **Intestinal Permeability and Its Relevance to Disease:** This review discusses the potential role of increased intestinal permeability in various diseases, highlighting the complex interplay with other factors.

Important Note:
While the research shows promising avenues, evidence directly linking general "gut leak" to specific symptoms and diseases remains limited. More research is needed to establish its validity and potential diagnostic methods.

If you experience concerning symptoms, it's crucial to consult a healthcare professional for an accurate diagnosis and appropriate treatment plans. Self-diagnosing and resorting to unproven interventions based on "gut leak" claims can be risky.

SCIENTIFIC TREATMENT FOR GUT LEAK: A NUANCE-FILLED LANDSCAPE

While the concept of "gut leak" has gained traction, its treatment remains complex and often contentious. The lack of a definitive diagnostic test and limited large-scale research create challenges in establishing standardized treatment protocols. Here's a breakdown of the current landscape:

Proposed Treatments:

- **Dietary Interventions:** These focus on gut-healing diets, typically emphasizing whole, unprocessed foods, increased fiber intake, and reduced inflammatory triggers like gluten or dairy. While some proponents tout their benefits, studies haven't definitively linked specific diets to reversing "gut leak."

- **Supplements:** Probiotics, glutamine (an amino acid), and various herbal remedies are often suggested, but evidence supporting their effectiveness for "gut leak" is limited or mixed.

- **Lifestyle Changes:** Stress management, sleep hygiene, and exercise are widely recognized to impact gut health, but their specific role in addressing "gut leak" requires further investigation.

Refuting Scientists and Concerns: Several scientists and medical professionals express skepticism about the concept of "gut leak" due to:

- The lack of standardized definitions and diagnostic criteria makes assessing the condition's existence and prevalence difficult.

- Limited high-quality research: Most studies investigating "gut leak" are small and lack robust evidence to establish specific treatments' validity and effectiveness.

- Focus on unproven interventions: Some approaches promoted for "gut leak" haven't undergone rigorous scientific evaluation and might raise safety concerns.

It's crucial to emphasize that:

- Self-diagnosing and treating "gut leak" based on online information can be dangerous. Consulting a qualified healthcare professional for proper diagnosis and evidence-based treatment plans is essential.

- Current research focuses on addressing underlying gut issues through healthy lifestyle choices and managing specific conditions associated with increased intestinal permeability.

Note: Always remember! Science is an ongoing process, and knowledge constantly evolves. Staying informed through reliable sources and consulting healthcare professionals ensures you make informed decisions regarding your health and well-being.

CHAPTER 35

TOOLBOX N36MRL BRAZILIAN RD VALMIRA CRISTINA DE ANDRADE

"Conhece-te a ti mesmo e conhecerás o universo e seus deuses /know thyself."

- Your purpose as a behavioral and emotional nutritionist is to transform the mental patterns of many people as possible. You aim to help people reprogram their minds to overcome unhealthy and obesogenic patterns and adopt healthy mental patterns, impacting their lives and helping them feel free, light, and happy.

- Through observation of people's mental patterns, behaviors, and feelings, you have understood that most live on autopilot, unaware of their emotions or actions, leading to erroneous eating behaviors and disastrous consequences.

- True happiness and health, you believe, come from eating only enough to live in balance—neither more nor less, but just enough.

- Upon realizing the importance of raising awareness, you discovered your purpose: to impact people's lives by helping them become conscious eaters. You aspire to reach everyone worldwide and guide them towards conscious eating habits.

- Envision a world where everyone eats consciously, in the right amount and quality! Diseases would be defeated, giving way to perfect health and quality of life.

- You aspire to have access to everyone in the world and teach them to observe the signs of hunger, satiety, and thirst that their bodies emit. You intend to introduce them to eating only when hungry and stopping when satiated. Additionally, you aim to teach them to be fully present in mind and body while eating, to eat slowly, savor their food, and chew thoroughly, preventing overeating, obesity, and related diseases.

- You believe people would be much happier if they ate the right way because their bodies would absorb more nutrients and be better nourished.

- From personal experience, you have observed instances of eating without necessity due to misinterpretation of feelings. Often, eating occurs when you need water, rest, or coping mechanisms for anxiety or emotion. Recognizing this behavior as standard, you aim to help people awaken their consciousness and diagnose their feelings before eating. This pre-eating self-questioning is crucial to prevent eating on autopilot and its consequences.

- You advocate that while food is pleasurable, it should never be the sole source of pleasure. People need to nourish themselves with other energies.

- In your vision, people would eat only when necessary, in adequate amounts, and in the proper manner. This intervention would challenge the food industry to reconsider its practices, which often prioritize profit over the health and lives of individuals, leading many to obesity and health complications.

- Consciousness, you believe, is the key to life, lightness, self-esteem, and longevity. Hence, it has become your mission and life purpose.

"And these lines awaken your consciousness, and your life will be nourished and healthy!"

CHAPTER 36

OBESITY: UNDERSTANDING THE COMPLEXITY, EMBRACING SUSTAINABLE SOLUTIONS

A Multifaceted Approach Exploring the Complexity of Obesity

This chapter moves beyond simplistic explanations of obesity, highlighting the multifaceted approach necessary for achieving and maintaining a healthy weight. Obesity, defined as having a body mass index (BMI) of 30 or higher, has become a global health crisis, impacting individuals and healthcare systems alike. But beneath this seemingly simple definition lies a multifaceted condition with diverse subtypes, complex causes, and nuanced approaches to management.

Unpacking the Diversity of Obesity:

While excess body fat is a common thread, recognizing different types of obesity is crucial for effective management. We can broadly categorize them as follows:

- **Visceral obesity:** Characterized by excess fat around internal organs, linked to increased risk of metabolic complications like type 2 diabetes and heart disease.

- **Subcutaneous obesity:** Primarily affects fat under the skin and has milder metabolic risks compared to visceral fat.

- **Secondary obesity:** Arises from underlying medical conditions like hormonal imbalances or medications.

Beyond Calories: Exploring the Etiology of Obesity:

While energy imbalance (consuming more calories than you burn) plays a role, obesity is not solely about willpower. Numerous factors contribute, including:

- **Genetics:** Certain gene variants predispose individuals to store more fat or regulate appetite less effectively.

- **Epigenetics:** Environmental factors during early development can impact gene expression, influencing obesity risk.

- **Gut microbiome:** Altered gut bacteria composition can affect nutrient absorption and metabolism, potentially contributing to weight gain.

- **Socioeconomic factors:** Food insecurity, limited access to healthy options, and stress can hinder healthy eating habits.

Navigating the Maze: Sustainable Approaches to Managing Obesity:

There is no magic bullet for obesity management. Instead, a multifaceted approach tailored to individual needs and preferences is crucial. Key components include:

- **Dietary interventions:** Focusing on whole, unprocessed foods, emphasizing fruits, vegetables, and whole grains while limiting processed foods and sugary drinks.

- **Physical activity:** Engaging in regular, moderate-intensity exercise to increase calorie expenditure and improve metabolic health.

- **Behavioral therapy:** Cognitive behavioral therapy can help address unhealthy eating habits and promote sustainable lifestyle changes.

- **Pharmacological therapy:** Medication under medical supervision may be considered alongside lifestyle changes for specific individuals.

THE IMPORTANCE OF A SAFE AND SUPPORTIVE ENVIRONMENT

Obesity management can be challenging, and individuals deserve a safe and supportive environment. This includes:

- **Combating weight stigma:** Stigma can perpetuate negative self-image and hinder motivation. Cultivating a culture of body acceptance and respect is crucial.

- **Addressing social determinants of health:** It is vital to ensure access to affordable, healthy food, safe neighborhoods for physical activity, and healthcare equity.

- **Promoting holistic well-being:** Recognizing the emotional and mental health aspects of obesity and providing accessible support systems.

Remember! Obesity is a complex issue; managing it requires a multifaceted approach. By understanding the different types, exploring contributing factors, and embracing sustainable, individual-centered strategies, we can move towards a healthier future for all.

Note: This information is for educational purposes only and should not be interpreted as medical advice. Please consult a healthcare professional for personalized guidance on managing obesity!

CHAPTER 37

TOOLBOX N639MRL: A JOURNEY TO MINDFUL OBESITY CONQUERING

For those at the junction of desiring transformation in their relationship with weight and body, a monumental journey awaits. This isn't a race nor a quick fix; it's a testament to discipline, self-exploration, and the gentle art of change. In this in-depth instructional guide, we'll embark on a 12-day journey tailored to the unique needs of those beginning their fight against the web of obesity and sedentary habits. It's about embracing a nutritional and fitness strategy that is not an act of endurance but a form of self-expression and self-liberation.

Day 1: The Art of Mindfulness in Your Eating Habits

Start the first day by understanding what it means to eat mindfully! It's about being present and conscious of every bite you take. Prepare your first meal without distractions: no phones, TV, or rushing! Take the time to savor textures, flavors, and the sensation of your body nourished by what you eat! This isn't just a meal; it's a practice of being in the moment, satiating your hunger while simultaneously training your mind to pay attention to your food.

Day 2: A Reflection Session

Set aside time to reflect on your feelings after yesterday's mindful meal! Notice the difference in satisfaction and apply this mindfulness to other areas of your life! Did you notice a change in energy levels? Perhaps a reduction in anxiety or stress? Use a journal to record these insights! The power of understanding the effect of your diet on your sense of well-being can be transformational.

Day 3: Mapping Your Food Consumption

Today, map out your food consumption! Notice patterns that may have been unconscious before and use this information to adjust where you see fit. Perhaps you're consuming more in the evenings or turning to a particular comfort food. Be kind to yourself in this discovery process! Knowledge is power, and awareness is the first step towards change.

Day 4: Establishing a Fitness Goal

Physical activity is vital. It's time to set a realistic fitness goal. Whether starting with a ten-minute walk or a beginner's yoga session, find a form of exercise that gives you joy! This isn't about punishment; it's about honoring your body with movement. Set an exciting goal, knowing every step counts towards your overall well-being!

Day 5: The Power of Habit Formation

Our lives are a collection of habits. Today, we focus on habit formation. Begin with a small yet pivotal habit, such as drinking more water daily. Consider acquiring an app that reminds you to drink a glass every hour! Understand the reward of satisfaction each time you complete this micro-goal, and let it inspire you to create other nourishing habits!

Day 6: Exploring a Nutrient-Dense Diet

Nutrition isn't about deprivation; it's about celebrating the vast array of nutrients nature offers. Explore different fruits, vegetables, whole grains, and lean proteins, and make at least one meal entirely from fresh, nutrient-dense foods. Notice how your body reacts to this high-quality fuel! Your energy levels may surge, and your mind may feel sharper.

Day 7: The Importance of Support and Community

Community is essential in any journey. Seek support from friends, family, or online groups! Share your experiences and learn from others! You might find solutions to common challenges or receive encouragement when it's needed the most. Remember! You are not alone on this journey.

Day 8: Crafting Your Ideal Fitness Routine

Use your experience from the past week's activities and observations to craft a fitness routine that aligns with your lifestyle and personal preferences! This routine should be both challenging and realistic. Find the time of day you feel most energetic and make that your fitness window! Whether it's early morning or late at night, consistency is critical.

Day 9: Overcoming Obstacles with Mindset Shifts

Today, uncover the hidden obstacles in your path! They could be mental or physical. Notice how specific thoughts or self-doubts can sabotage your best intentions! Practice mindset shifts to overcome these obstacles! Affirmations, visualizations, or positive self-talk can turn those stumbling blocks into stepping stones.

Day 10: Revitalizing Through Rest and Recovery

Rest and recovery are as critical as activity. Today, focus on revitalizing your body through proper rest! Aim for 7-9 hours of quality sleep and engage in activities that promote relaxation, such as deep breathing exercises or a soothing bath. Remember, your body rejuvenates during rest, which is fundamental to a balanced, active life.

Day 11: The Interplay of Mind and Body

The interplay of mind and body is profound. Engage in an activity that challenges your body and enriches your mind! It could be a yoga class focusing on mindfulness, a hike where you can appreciate the beauty around you, or a meditation connecting your physical and mental states.

Day 12: Celebrating Progress and Setting New Goals

As you approach the end of this 12-day journey, take time to celebrate your progress! Acknowledge the changes, no matter how small they may seem! Every step you've taken is a step in the right direction. Use this positivity to set new goals that continue building on your achievements! Remember! This is a journey of continuous growth and self-discovery.

Genuine transformation can begin by taking this 12-day journey with dedicated intention. It's a journey of self-examination, recognizing patterns and new habits, and celebrating every breakthrough. Embracing the process with radical acceptance and love for oneself is at the heart of conquering obesity and nurturing a healthy, fulfilling life.

Remember, consistency is key! Please choose a method that fits your lifestyle and stick with it for a few weeks to see patterns emerge!

The beauty of tracking:

It's not about restrictions but about self-discovery. As you track across different countries, you'll learn.

CHAPTER 38

NAVIGATING HEALTH WITH SPECIAL NEEDS

WHY REGISTERED DIETITIANS ARE ESSENTIAL FOR SPECIAL POPULATIONS AND CHRONIC DISEASES

Navigating the world of nutrition can be daunting for individuals with special populations and chronic diseases. Their dietary needs differ vastly from those of the general population, and managing them alongside specific health conditions necessitates expert guidance. This is where registered dietitians (RDs) step in, playing a vital role in optimizing their health and well-being.

Understanding the Unique Needs:

Special Populations: Children, pregnant women, older adults, and individuals with disabilities have specific nutritional requirements that differ from the general population. RDs possess the expertise to tailor dietary plans to meet these unique needs, promoting growth, development, and overall health.

Chronic Diseases: Conditions like diabetes, heart disease, kidney disease, and cancer often necessitate specific dietary modifications to manage symptoms, prevent complications, and improve quality of life. RDs are trained to understand the intricacies of these conditions and translate them into practical, personalized dietary interventions.

The Power of Collaboration:

RDs collaborate with physicians, nurses, and other healthcare professionals to develop comprehensive treatment plans. This collaborative approach ensures that nutritional needs are addressed alongside other medical interventions, optimizing health outcomes.

Benefits of Registered Dietitian Support:

- **Improved Disease Management:** RDs can design personalized meal plans that help manage blood sugar levels, blood pressure, and other disease-specific parameters.

- **Reduced Risk of Complications:** By optimizing nutrition, RDs can help individuals with chronic diseases reduce their risk of further complications.

- **Enhanced Quality of Life:** RDs can empower individuals to make informed food choices, promote energy levels, manage symptoms, and improve overall well-being.

- **Personalized Guidance:** RDs consider individual preferences, cultural needs, and lifestyle factors to create sustainable and enjoyable dietary plans.

- **Evidence-based Approach:** RDs base their recommendations on scientific evidence and stay up-to-date on the latest research in nutrition and specific disease management.

Why Prioritizing RD Support is Crucial:

For individuals with special populations and chronic diseases, access to RD support is not just beneficial. It's essential. It can:

- **Reduce Healthcare Costs:** By preventing complications and promoting better management, RDs can help reduce the burden on healthcare systems.

- **Empower Individuals:** RDs equip individuals with the knowledge and skills to manage their health, fostering self-advocacy and independence.

- **Promote Community Well-being:** By addressing the needs of special populations and individuals with chronic diseases, RDs contribute to a healthier and more vibrant community.

In Conclusion, registered dietitians are invaluable partners for individuals with special needs and chronic diseases on their journey toward optimal health and well-being. Investing in RD support is not just a matter of individual benefit but a crucial step towards creating a healthier, more empowered community.

CHAPTER 39

BUILDING YOUR SUPPORT SYSTEM: THE POWER OF COLLABORATION

Beyond individual effort, this chapter emphasizes the importance of building a supportive network of healthcare professionals, loved ones, and communities to contribute to your overall well-being.

FOOD ALLERGIES AND POISONING: RECOGNIZING THREATS TO WELL-BEING

Food allergies and poisoning pose distinct yet significant threats to well-being, necessitating both proactive avoidance and prompt intervention. This guide delves into these critical topics, equipping you with scientific knowledge and actionable strategies.

Recognizing Food Allergies:

Immune Response: Food allergies trigger an exaggerated immune reaction upon exposure to specific allergens, such as peanuts or shellfish.

Symptoms: Manifestations can vary across individuals, but common reactions include:

- **Cutaneous:** Urticaria (hives), angioedema (swelling), eczema.

- **Gastrointestinal:** Nausea, vomiting, abdominal pain, diarrhea.

- **Respiratory:** Wheezing, shortness of breath, anaphylaxis (life-threatening).

- **Cardiovascular:** Dizziness, hypotension, syncope.

Anaphylaxis: Immediate medical attention is crucial, as untreated anaphylaxis can be fatal.

Seeking Professional Support:

- **Allergy Testing:** Accurate diagnosis is paramount. Consult a board-certified allergist for a comprehensive evaluation, including a detailed history, physical examination, and skin prick or blood tests.

- **Dietary Management:** To avoid allergens, it is crucial to follow a strict elimination diet guided by an allergist or registered dietitian.

- **Emergency Preparedness:** Carry an epinephrine auto-injector (e.g., EpiPen) prescribed by your allergist, and wear a medical alert bracelet.

- **Psychological Support:** Living with allergies can be stressful. Consider seeking counseling to manage anxiety and promote emotional well-being.

Preventing Food Poisoning:

Foodborne Pathogens: Bacterial (e.g., Salmonella), viral (e.g., norovirus), or parasitic (e.g., Giardia) contamination can cause food poisoning.

High-Risk Foods: Undercooked meat, poultry, seafood, unpasteurized dairy products, and improperly handled fruits and vegetables pose an increased risk.

Safe Food Handling Practices:

- **Clean:** Wash hands and surfaces thoroughly before, during, and after food preparation.

- **Separate:** Avoid cross-contamination using separate cutting boards and utensils for raw and cooked foods.

- **Cook:** Use a food thermometer to ensure proper internal cooking temperatures for meat, poultry, and eggs.

- **Chill:** Refrigerate or freeze leftovers promptly within two hours of cooking.

- **Thaw:** Thaw frozen foods safely in the refrigerator or under cold running water.

International Studies and Articles:
- *The Lancet:* Global Burden of Disease Study 2019 - estimated foodborne illness contributes to over 420,000 deaths annually.

- *Journal of Allergy and Clinical Immunology:* Food Allergies: A Global Epidemic - highlights the rising prevalence of food allergies worldwide.

- *World Health Organization:* Food Safety - provides evidence-based guidance on preventing foodborne diseases.

Disclaimer:

This information is intended for educational purposes only and should not be construed as medical advice. Always consult a healthcare professional for diagnosis and treatment of food allergies and food poisoning.

Remember! Vigilance in recognizing allergic reactions, seeking professional guidance, and adhering to safe food handling practices are crucial in navigating the food labyrinth and safeguarding your health.

CHAPTER 40

FITNESS: UNLEASH YOUR POTENTIAL!
"Fitness ain't about punishment; it's about reclaiming."

Before we embark on this modern fitness adventure, let's travel back in time, imagining our ancestors who embraced movement as a way of life! Fast-forward to today, when we're bombarded with fitness trends and marketing hype. But the truth is, fitness is about reclaiming your body's power, the joy of movement, and the confidence that radiates from within. It's not about punishment; it's about progress. Progress in strength, energy, and overall well-being.

If you're ready to ditch the pain-driven approach and embrace a movement that feels good, both physically and mentally, then buckle up! This isn't your grandma's workout routine. We blend ancient wisdom with modern technology to create a personalized, robust, sustainable fitness experience. So, let's rewrite the fitness narrative and embark on a journey towards your best self! Are you ready? Let's go!

Lorenzi R.Marcos

A SYMPHONY OF LIFE: EXPLORING THE MARVELS OF THE HUMAN BODY

"The human body is the greatest masterpiece of nature." - Michelangelo.

The human body is a marvel of interconnected systems, each performing a delicate dance of life. Let's delve into some quantifiable wonders that make us who we are!

Remember! These numbers represent only glimpses into the vastness of the human body. As we marvel at its quantifiable aspects, let us also appreciate the resilience of the human spirit and the boundless potential within each of us!

May this exploration empower you to appreciate the incredible gift of your own body, a symphony of life playing out in every breath, every beat, and every thought!

YES, it's not a simple question of how to be in shape; it's how to be healthy. Let's explore further how we can operate this machine at its highest performance before crafting a fitness routine without leaving behind fear, shame, and regrets!

CHAPTER 41

30 PHYSICAL ACTIVITIES: UNLEASH YOUR POTENTIAL WITH SCIENCE-BACKED BENEFITS

Here's a diverse list of 30 physical activities, categorized by training concepts and their associated benefits, along with scientific references and recommendations for different age groups:

Power:

1. **Box Jumping:** Improves explosive leg power and vertical jump. (Reference: Journal of Strength and Conditioning Research)
   Recommendation: Ages 18-45 with proper form and guidance.

2. **Olympic Weightlifting:** Develops total body power and explosiveness. (Reference: Sports Medicine)
   Recommendation: Ages 18+ with qualified coaching due to technical complexity.

3. **Medicine Ball Slams:** Enhance rotational power and core stability. (Reference: International Journal of Sports Physiology and Performance)
   Recommendation: Ages 16+, with proper form and lighter weights for beginners.

4. **Plyometrics:** Builds explosive power and speed through jump variations. (Reference: Journal of Athletic Training)
   Recommendation: Ages 16+ with good baseline fitness and an injury prevention focus.

Strength:

5. **Bodyweight Exercises (Push-ups, Squats, Lunges):** Builds functional strength with minimal equipment. (Reference: American College of Sports Medicine)
   Recommendation: All ages with modifications for different fitness levels.

6. **Weight Training:** Progressive overload with free weights or machines builds targeted muscle strength. (Reference: National Strength and Conditioning Association)
   Recommendation: For all ages, especially beginners, with proper form and supervision.

7. **Resistance Bands:** Versatile and portable tools for strength training at home or on the go. (Reference: ACSM Health & Fitness Journal)
   Recommendation: All ages with appropriate resistance levels.

8. **Climbing (Rock Climbing, Bouldering):** Builds upper body and grip strength while challenging coordination and problem-solving. (Reference: Journal of Sports Sciences)
   Recommendation: All ages with appropriate supervision and climbing gyms catering to different skill levels.

Endurance:

9. **Running:** A classic cardio exercise for improving cardiovascular health and endurance. (Reference: Progress in Cardiovascular Diseases)
   Recommendation: All ages with appropriate pacing and footwear.

10. **Swimming:** A low-impact, full-body workout that improves cardiovascular health and endurance. (Reference: Sports Medicine)
    Recommendation: All ages with proper aquatic safety skills.

11. **Cycling:** Builds leg strength and endurance while offering scenic outdoor options. (Reference: British Journal of Sports Medicine)
    Recommendation: All ages with appropriate bicycles and safety measures.

12. **Dancing:** A fun and social activity that improves cardiovascular health, endurance, and coordination. (Reference: International Journal of Dance)
    Recommendation: All ages and with various dance styles.

Hypertrophy (Muscle Growth):

13. **Weight Training (Heavy Loads):** Progressive overload with heavier weights stimulates muscle growth. (Reference: The American Journal of Physiology)
    Recommendation: Ages 18+ with proper form and focus on compound exercises.

14. **Bodybuilding Routines:** Specific sets and rep ranges tailored for muscle growth. (Reference: Strength & Conditioning Journal)
    Recommendation: Ages 18+ with experience and knowledge of training principles.

15. **Powerlifting:** Lifting maximal weights for one repetition builds size and strength simultaneously. (Reference: Journal of Strength and Conditioning Research)
    Recommendation: Ages 18+ with advanced training experience and coaching.

16. **Calisthenics (Advanced Movements):** Bodyweight exercises with progressions challenge muscles for growth. (Reference: Sports Medicine)
    Recommendation: Advanced athletes with a strong foundation in bodyweight movements.

Weight Loss:

17. **HIIT (High-Intensity Interval Training):** Burn calories efficiently through alternating high-intensity and recovery periods. (Reference: Medicine & Science in Sports & Exercise)
    Recommendation: All ages with modifications for fitness levels and consultation with healthcare professionals if needed.

Flexibility and Mobility:

18. **Yoga:** Improves flexibility, balance, and core strength while reducing stress. (Reference: International Journal of Yoga)
Recommendation: All ages, with modifications for different levels.

19. **Tai Chi:** Gentle movements enhance flexibility, balance, and posture, promoting relaxation and mindfulness. (Reference: The Cochrane Database of Systematic Reviews)
Recommendation: All ages.

20. **Pilates:** Low-impact exercises that improve flexibility, core strength, and posture, with variations for different fitness levels. (Reference: Journal of Bodywork and Movement Therapies)
Recommendation: All ages with modifications for various levels.

Balance and Coordination:

21. **Dancing (Specific Styles):** Styles like ballet, ballroom, or line dancing require precise movements, improving balance and coordination. (Reference: Journal of Sport and Rehabilitation)
Recommendation: All ages with appropriate styles.

22. **Martial Arts:** Karate, Taekwondo, or Judo offer physical conditioning while developing balance, coordination, and self-defense skills. (Reference: The Physician and Sportsmedicine)
Recommendation: All ages with modifications for different fitness levels.

23. **Agility Ladder Drills:** Footwork drills using a ladder improve agility, coordination, and speed. (Reference: Journal of Strength and Conditioning Research)
Recommendation: All ages with modifications for fitness levels.

Mental Well-being:

24. **Hiking:** Immersing yourself in nature reduces stress and anxiety while providing moderate exercise. (Reference: Environmental Science & Technology)
    Recommendation: All ages with appropriate trails and precautions.

25. **Rock Climbing (Guided Tours):** Challenging climbs can be mentally stimulating and build confidence, especially on guided tours for beginners. (Reference: Journal of Outdoor Recreation and Education)
    Recommendation: All ages should have proper instruction and safety measures.

26. **Team Sports:** Playing basketball, soccer, or volleyball provides physical activity and social interaction and can reduce stress. (Reference: Social Science & Medicine)
    Recommendation: All ages with modifications for different fitness levels and abilities.

Overall Fitness and Fun:

27. **Circuit Training:** Combining various exercises with short rest periods provides a full-body workout and improves cardiovascular health. (Reference: The American College of Sports Medicine)
    Recommendation: All ages with modifications for fitness levels.

28. **Rowing:** This low-impact, full-body exercise engages significant muscle groups and improves cardiovascular health. (Reference: Sports Medicine)
    Recommendation: Proper technique and supervision are recommended for all ages.

29. **Sports (Recreational):** Playing tennis, badminton, or frisbee offers fun, social interaction, and moderate exercise. (Reference: Journal of Physical Activity and Health)
    Recommendation: All ages with modifications for different fitness levels and abilities.

30. **Swimming (Specific Activities):** Water aerobics or synchronized swimming add variety and challenge to regular swimming, improving fitness and coordination. (Reference: Journal of Strength and Conditioning Research)
Recommendation: All ages with proper aquatic safety skills.

Remember! These are just suggestions. You can choose activities that best suit your interests, fitness level, and goals.

Disclaimer: This information is intended for educational purposes only and should not be substituted for professional medical advice. Always consult with a healthcare professional before starting any new exercise program!

CHAPTER 42

RISE, BREAK FREE: UNLEASH YOUR POTENTIAL BEYOND THE NOISE!

I stare back at you from the mirror – skinny, unassuming, the antithesis of the sculpted figures plastered across marketing billboards. The voice whispers, "You're not built for this," echoes of bias fueling self-doubt. But here I stand, a certified personal trainer, living proof that the fitness industry's narrow narrative is a lie.

My journey began in the same place you might be now – hesitant, intimidated, and lost in the maze of unrealistic expectations. Yet, within me burned a spark, a yearning to defy limitations fueled by the wisdom of stoicism. Like Gandhi's unwavering spirit, I refused to react, instead choosing to take control, not of the noise, but of my transformation.

My approach? Empathy, not judgment. I've witnessed countless others grapple with the same self-doubt, their potential shackled by the industry's distorted image. But beneath the perceived "limitations" lies a universe waiting to be explored.

This isn't just about sculpted bodies; it's about sculpting minds and souls. Fitness is your canvas, a brush in your hand to paint strength, resilience, and self-belief. Forget the external pressures, the comparisons, the voices of limitation. This journey is yours, fueled by your unique fire.

Please don't listen to the noise, don't react to the limitations, rise above them, and embrace the process, the stumbles, and the triumphs! You sculpt your physique, confidence, and spirit in every step, rep.

I stand before you, not as the epitome of perfection, but as a testament to possibility. Break free from the confines of what you think you can't achieve! Remember! The most extraordinary transformation begins not with your body but with your mind. It starts with believing in yourself, owning your canvas, and painting a masterpiece called you.

Together, let's rewrite the narrative! Let's rise, more muscular, accessible, and empowered, not just physically, but in the truest sense of the word!

CHAPTER 43

YOUR FITNESS JOURNEY: A SCIENCE-BASED APPROACH

Starting a fitness journey can be both exciting and overwhelming. To ensure a safe and successful experience, consider these steps, incorporating biomechanics, postural deviations, and any unique health concerns:

Seek Professional Guidance:
- Consult a healthcare professional: Before starting any new exercise program, especially if you have pre-existing health conditions, undergo a physical examination and get clearance from a doctor or physiotherapist! They can identify potential limitations and tailor a plan that prioritizes your safety and individual needs.

- Find a qualified fitness professional: A certified personal trainer or exercise coach can assess your biomechanics, posture, and fitness level, design a personalized program, and provide guidance on proper form and technique to minimize injury risk.

Build a Strong Foundation:
- Focus on basic movement patterns: Master fundamental movements like squats, lunges, pushes, pulls, and core exercises using good form before progressing to more complex training. This strengthens your foundation and reduces the risk of injury.

- Address postural deviations: If you have postural imbalances, incorporate corrective exercises and stretches recommended by your healthcare professional or fitness coach. Addressing these imbalances can improve movement efficiency and prevent pain.

- Prioritize mobility and flexibility: Regularly perform dynamic stretches and drills to improve your range of motion and joint health. This allows for better exercise execution and injury prevention.

Lorenzi R.Marcos

Tailor Your Training to Your Goals and Needs:
- Define your goals: Weight loss, muscle gain, improved cardiovascular health, or overall fitness. Knowing your goals helps you select appropriate exercises and training modalities.

- Choose activities you enjoy: Engage in fun and sustainable activities to increase adherence to the program! Explore different options like walking, swimming, dancing, yoga, or team sports!

- Start gradually and progress safely: Begin with lower intensity and volume, progressively increasing difficulty and duration as your fitness improves! Listen to your body and avoid pushing yourself too hard, too soon!

Embrace a Holistic Approach:
- Prioritize sleep: Aim for 7-8 hours of quality sleep each night! Sleep is crucial for muscle recovery, energy levels, and overall health, impacting your fitness journey significantly.

- Fuel your body correctly: Eat a nutritious diet rich in fruits, vegetables, whole grains, and lean protein to give your body the nutrients it needs for optimal performance and recovery!

- Manage stress: Chronic stress can hinder your progress. Practice stress-management techniques like meditation, yoga, or spending time in nature to promote well-being and support your fitness goals!

International Guidance:
- The World Health Organization (WHO): WHO recommends that adults engage in at least 150 minutes of moderate-intensity aerobic activity or 75 minutes of vigorous-intensity aerobic activity per week, along with muscle-strengthening exercises two or more days per week.

- American College of Sports Medicine (ACSM): This organization provides similar recommendations, emphasizing gradual progression, individualization, and adherence to safety guidelines.

Remember: Consistency is critical. By following these science-based steps and prioritizing your personal needs, you can embark on a safe and sustainable fitness journey that empowers you to reach your goals and experience the joy of movement.

Disclaimer: This information is for educational purposes only and should not be substituted for professional medical or fitness advice. Always consult with a healthcare professional before starting any new exercise program!

CHAPTER 44

A SCIENCE-GUIDED APPROACH TO YOUR FITNESS JOURNEY PART 2

Now that we've established the crucial prerequisites for a safe and successful fitness journey let's delve into the heart of the action – the training program itself! Buckle up as we explore each phase with friendly encouragement and professional insights while recognizing the uniqueness of individual needs and potential health considerations!

Stretching:
- Static stretches held for 20-30 seconds each target major muscle groups and areas relevant to your chosen activity.

- Stretching an astonishing muscle is more effective and reduces the risk of injury than stretching a warm muscle.

- Stretching prepares your muscles for movement and improves flexibility, enhancing performance and range of motion.

Warming Up:
- Gentle movements like dynamic stretches, light cardio, and joint rotations activate your muscles, elevate your heart rate, and increase blood flow.

- This prepares your body for more intense activity in Phase 3 and minimizes the risk of injury.

- Consider dynamic stretches that mimic the movements you will be doing in your workout for optimal preparation!

Conditioning:
- This phase includes cardio, strength training, and mobility/flexibility drills tailored to your individual goals and needs.

- Remember, listen to your body, start gradually, and progress safely!

Cooldown:

- Light cardio, static stretches held for longer durations (30-60 seconds), and deep breathing help your body wind down and recover properly.

- This reduces post-workout soreness and promotes overall well-being.

Remember! This is a general guideline. Always consult a healthcare professional or qualified fitness coach for personalized advice based on your circumstances!

CHAPTER 45

THE FITNESS CROSSROADS: GYM VS. HOME FOR BEGINNERS

Congratulations on embarking on this incredible journey of self-discovery and transformation through fitness! Whether you're a beginner or rediscovering movement after a break, choosing between a gym and home workouts can feel overwhelming. Fear not! This guide will illuminate the pros and cons of each path, empower you with exploration possibilities, and equip you with key points for an optimal decision.

The Gym Arena:
Pros:

- Equipment galore: Access to diverse machines, weights, and tools for targeted workouts.

- Community vibes: Meet like-minded individuals, get motivated by group classes, and feel the energy of shared goals.

- Expert guidance: Certified trainers can personalize programs, correct forms, and answer questions.

- Structured environment: A space dedicated to exercise, minimizing distractions.

Cons:

- Cost factor: Monthly fees can add up, especially with personal training sessions.

- Travel time: Commuting eats into workout time and adds logistical hurdles.

- Crowds and schedules: Equipment wait times and class timings can limit flexibility.

- Intimidation factor: Gyms can feel overwhelming for newbies, hindering enjoyment.

Home Turf:

Pros:

- Comfort and convenience: Work out in your pajamas, at your own pace, whenever suits you.

- Cost-effective: Minimal or no equipment needed, eliminating gym fees.

- Privacy and flexibility: No crowds, distractions, or judgmental eyes.

- Personalized focus: Tailor workouts to your specific needs and preferences.

Cons:

- Limited equipment: Might lack tools for targeted muscle groups or advanced training.

- Motivation matters: Requires self-discipline to stay consistent without the external push.

- Distraction zone: The home environment can tempt you to multitask or skip workouts.

- Technical guidance: Mastering form and progression alone can be challenging.

Explore Your Fitness Landscape:

- Take free gym trials: Experience the equipment, atmosphere, and classes firsthand!

- Browse online home workout programs: Find free routines or subscribe to affordable platforms!

- Seek fitness buddy support: Partner with a friend or family member for accountability and motivation!

- Consider hybrid options: Combine gym sessions with home workouts for a flexible approach!

The Key Decision:
Ultimately, the "best" choice depends on your needs, personality, and lifestyle. Do you thrive in structured environments or relish personalized flexibility? Are cost and convenience significant factors? Listen to your intuition and choose the path that sparks your enthusiasm and feels sustainable in the long run!

NEUROSCIENCE AND THE POWER OF CHOICE

Remember, exercise doesn't just sculpt your body; it rewires your brain for resilience and joy! Studies show that physical activity releases endorphins, boosts mood, and enhances cognitive function. So, celebrate your decision, regardless of gym or home, knowing you're investing in your mental and physical well-being!

Your Freedom to Inspire:

This is more than just about choosing a workout space; it's about claiming freedom to move, explore, and transform. Your journey inspires others, demonstrating the power of taking the first step towards a healthier, happier you. So, embrace this adventure with optimism, knowing you're not just changing yourself but potentially inspiring positive change around you!

The most important decision is to start moving. Choose the path that feels right for you, and enjoy the incredible journey of self-discovery and empowerment that awaits you!

Reference:

1. Global Report on Physical Activity 2022 by the World Health Organization (WHO): The Global Status Report on Physical Activity 2022 (who. int)

2. "The Dose-Response Relationship Between Physical Activity and Health: A Review and Critical Evaluation" published in the British Journal of Sports Medicine (2018): Physical activity— maximizing benefits for all | British Journal of Sports Medicine (bmj.com)

3. "Physical Activity and Mental Health" published in the Lancet Psychiatry (2018): Physical activity and mental health - The Lancet Psychiatry

By presenting these studies, I aim to illustrate the undeniable scientific evidence supporting the significant benefits of physical activity, regardless of your chosen environment. Whether you exercise at home or the gym, the key message is to start moving and commit to regular physical activity to reap the countless rewards for your physical and mental well-being. Remember, every step towards a healthier lifestyle counts!

CHAPTER 46

SCIENCE-BASED EXERCISE PRESCRIPTION: TAILORING WORKOUTS FOR YOUR GOALS

As a certified personal trainer, I understand the importance of designing exercise programs based on individual goals and scientific principles. This guide dives into the vital exercise categories. It explains optimizing their frequency, intensity, time/volume, and progression for various fitness aims: weight loss, muscle gain, strength, power, speed, and endurance. Consulting a healthcare professional before starting any new program is crucial, especially if you have health concerns.

Exercise Categories:

- **Cardio:** Improves cardiovascular health and endurance and aids in weight management.

- **Strength Training:** Builds muscle mass, increases strength, and enhances bone density.

- **Flexibility:** Improves range of motion, reduces injury risk, and promotes good posture.

- **Balance:** Enhances stability and coordination and prevents falls.

SCIENCE-BASED RECOMMENDATIONS

Frequency:

- **Cardio:** Aim for 150-300 minutes of moderate-intensity cardio or 75-150 minutes of vigorous-intensity cardio per week (ACSM).

- **Strength Training:** 2-4 non-consecutive weekly sessions targeting all major muscle groups (ACSM).

- **Flexibility:** At least 2-3 weekly sessions, holding stretches for 20-30 seconds each (NSCA).

- **Balance:** Include balance exercises most days of the week, even for just a few minutes (ACSM).

Intensity:

- **Cardio:** Use methods like RPE (Rate of Perceived Exertion) or percentage of heart rate max to target moderate or vigorous intensity based on your goal.

- **Strength Training:** Choose weights that challenge you for 8-12 repetitions (muscle gain) or 1-6 repetitions (strength) with good form.

- **Flexibility:** Focus on smooth, controlled movements without bouncing.

- **Balance:** Start with simple exercises like single-leg stands and progress to more challenging drills.

Time/Volume:

- **Cardio:** For beginners, start with shorter durations and gradually increase. 30-minute sessions are a good starting point.

- **Strength Training:** Beginners can start with 2-3 sets of 8-12 repetitions per exercise. Aim for a total workout time of 30-60 minutes.

- **Flexibility:** Hold each stretch for 20-30 seconds and repeat 2-3 times! Aim for a total flexibility session of 15-20 minutes.

- **Balance:** Start with short 5-minute sessions and gradually increase duration and difficulty.

Lorenzi R.Marcos

Progression:

- Gradually increase frequency, intensity, time/volume, or exercise difficulty as you adapt and progress.

- Listen to your body and rest when needed to avoid injury or overtraining.Tailoring to Your Goals:

- **Weight Loss:** Prioritize cardio with moderate-intensity workouts lasting 45-60 minutes! Include strength training 2-3 times per week to preserve muscle mass.

- **Muscle Gain:** Focus on strength training with higher intensity (heavy weights, 8-12 reps) and higher volume (3-4 sets per exercise), and ensure adequate protein intake.

- **Strength:** Prioritize exercises with low reps (1-6) and heavier weights! Focus on compound exercises that work for multiple muscle groups.

- **Power:** Combine strength training with explosive movements like plyometrics and Olympic lifts, and practice quick sprints and power drills.

- **Speed:** Short bursts of high-intensity training (HIIT) combined with agility drills and sprints are essential. Strength training is also crucial for power development.

- **Endurance:** Focus on longer-duration cardio activities like running, swimming, or cycling at moderate intensity, gradually increasing distance and duration.

Remember! This is a general overview. Seek professional guidance for a personalized program considering your fitness level, health, and specific goals! Stay active, stay informed, and enjoy the journey towards a healthier you!

Disclaimer: This information is intended for educational purposes only and should not be interpreted as personalized medical advice. Always consult with a healthcare professional before starting any new exercise program!

CHAPTER 47

BREATHING FOR SUCCESS: OPTIMIZING OXYGEN FLOW DURING EXERCISE

Breathing, often relegated to the background during exercise, is crucial in optimizing performance and preventing injury. Understanding proper breathing techniques and recognizing warning signs for cessation is essential for a safe and productive workout.

The Mechanics of Breath:
During exercise, the demand for oxygen increases. The diaphragm, a dome-shaped muscle below the lungs, contracts, expanding the chest cavity and allowing air to enter. Conversely, relaxation of the diaphragm facilitates exhale. Effective breathing utilizes the diaphragm and intercostal muscles between the ribs, maximizing air intake and expulsion.

Best Practices for Exercise Breathing:
- **Nasal and Diaphragmatic Breathing:** Engage the diaphragm for deep, controlled breaths primarily through the nose, ensuring efficient oxygen delivery and minimizing unnecessary energy expenditure! Mouth breathing may be employed during intense bouts for additional air intake.

- **Rhythm and Pattern:** Maintain a consistent breathing pattern in sync with your movements! For example, breathe in for two steps during jogging and exhale for the next two. Avoid holding your breath, as this restricts oxygen availability and limits performance!

Warning Signs for Cessation:
- **Sharp Chest Pain or Discomfort:** Discontinue exercise immediately and seek medical attention! This could indicate a cardiac issue.

- **Severe Shortness of Breath:** If breathing becomes labored and significantly restricts activity, gradually stop and rest! If symptoms persist, consult a healthcare professional!

- **Lightheadedness or Dizziness:** These may indicate inadequate oxygen supply. Stop exercising, sit or lie down, and monitor your condition! If symptoms worsen, seek medical attention!

- **Excessive Wheezing or Coughing:** If coughing or wheezing becomes severe, particularly in individuals with asthma or allergies, cease exercise and use inhalers if prescribed! Consult a healthcare professional if symptoms persist!

- **Extreme Fatigue or Muscle Aches:** While fatigue is expected during exercise, excessive tiredness or unusual muscle aches may indicate overexertion. Rest and gradually resume activity after recovery!

Remember! Listen to your body and prioritize safety! Seek professional guidance if you are unsure about breathing techniques or experience any concerning symptoms during exercise. By understanding proper breathing practices and recognizing warning signs, you can optimize your workouts and perform at your best.

Disclaimer: *This information is intended for educational purposes only and should not be interpreted as personalized medical advice. Always consult a healthcare professional before starting any new exercise program or experiencing concerning symptoms during activity.*

CHAPTER 48

CASE STUDIES
Mr. Umar Arif's Journey as a Fitness Coach

Like many peers, I graduated with a business degree, but a more profound calling steered me away from the corporate world. I sensed that my purpose lay beyond profit-driven ventures; I wanted a direct impact on people's lives.

From my high school days, I harbored a passion for exercise and fitness. Encouraged by this passion, I decided to chart my career path as a fitness professional. I owe a debt of gratitude to my mother, whose support enabled me to finance my first fitness trainer certification.

However, my journey began at a sluggish pace. Initially, I had just one client whom I trained at their home post-certification. Although I secured a second client soon after, setbacks followed as my first client relocated for work. I grappled with minimal income for a year and a half, contemplating abandoning my aspirations as gym opportunities were scarce and poorly remunerated.

Exploring teaching as an alternative career, I encountered overwhelming stress, leading to severe health issues and my eventual resignation in November 2019. Despite these setbacks, I persisted in training a solitary client and expanding my exercise science and nutrition knowledge.

The onset of the COVID-19 pandemic presented further challenges, but with unwavering support from my parents, I transitioned to online training. In May 2021, a breakthrough arrived when I was recruited by a premier gym in my city, marking a pivotal juncture in my professional journey. My previous teaching experience proved invaluable in my evolution as a coach.

Today, I stand as a testament to resilience, determination, and a genuine dedication to empowering others through fitness. Believing staunchly in exercise's transformative potential, I endeavor to inspire individuals to embrace healthier lifestyles.

My growth owes much to the guidance of mentors such as Dr. Mike Israetel, Dr. Brad Schoenfeld, Bret Contreras, Dr. Layne Norton, and Dr. Eric Helms, whose profound insights have profoundly shaped my coaching philosophy.

CHAPTER 49

WHAT CHANGES WOULD I LIKE TO SEE IN THE FITNESS INDUSTRY?

Once rooted in the noble pursuit of aiding individuals in their health journey, the fitness industry is now increasingly driven by capitalist motives. Unfortunately, prioritizing clients' well-being often takes a backseat to pursuing monetary gains.

Furthermore, the sports supplement industry has capitalized on people's aspirations for enhanced physical performance and health. However, in doing so, it needs to pay more attention to the core value of addressing individuals' actual needs.

In addition, certifying agencies within the fitness industry prioritize profit generation over ensuring high-quality education for aspiring coaches. As a fitness educator, I have encountered instances where course content needs to align with the latest research, highlighting systemic issues in educational standards.

Moreover, the focus on fitness certifications and education has shifted towards accumulating continuing education units rather than a genuine quest for valuable knowledge to better serve clients.

I advocate for a fundamental shift in mindset among fitness professionals. Unless the industry reorients its focus to prioritize the well-being and needs of individuals, it risks straying further from its essential purpose.

CHAPTER 50

NAVIGATING THE LABYRINTH OF THE MIND

The intricacies of the human mind, with its myriad thoughts, emotions, and disorders, can be profoundly perplexing. In this exploration, we embark on a journey through emotional and mental disorders, recognizing the diverse spectrum of presentations individuals may encounter. We delve into the influences of environment, genetics, and epigenetics on mental health, acknowledging the evolutionary echoes reverberating within our psyche.

Emotional and Mental Disorders

Understanding emotional and mental disorders is pivotal in navigating the labyrinth of the mind. From anxiety to personality disorders, each condition presents unique challenges. By providing an overview of common diagnoses, we equip readers with the knowledge to identify and comprehend the experiences of those affected.

Spectrum of Presentations

Mental health manifests along a spectrum, varying in severity and symptomatology for each individual. By acknowledging the breadth of presentations, readers can better provide support and seek appropriate treatment pathways.

Environment, Genetics, Epigenetics

The interplay between environmental and genetic factors shapes mental health outcomes. We explore this complex relationship, highlighting potential triggers and protective factors influencing mental well-being.

Addiction

Addiction poses a significant challenge to mental health. We delve into its biological, psychological, and social underpinnings, offering insights to guide individuals toward recovery and support.

Evolutionary Echoes

Understanding the echoes of human evolution elucidates our psychological makeup and behaviors. By addressing these deep-rooted patterns, we can more effectively navigate the complexities of modern life.

Support for Loved Ones

Support from friends and family is crucial in mental health recovery. To provide practical assistance, we outline effective strategies, emphasizing communication and empathy.

Lifestyle Choices

Lifestyle factors profoundly impact mental health. Readers are empowered to make informed decisions regarding diet, exercise, and sleep habits, fostering improved well-being.

Stigma

The stigma surrounding mental health creates barriers to support and recovery. We examine its sources and impact, advocating for a more inclusive and supportive environment.

Understanding and Action

Empowering individuals to advocate for their mental health is paramount. We detail strategies for accessing resources and collaborating with mental health professionals, facilitating successful recovery.

The Symphony of Sustenance

The relationship between nutrition and mental health is explored, recognizing diet as a fundamental aspect of well-being. International studies highlight the impact of dietary choices on mental health outcomes.

Poor Nutrition

Inadequate dietary choices can exacerbate mental health conditions. We examine the links between poor nutrition and disorders such as depression and anxiety.

Mental Health Degeneration
Nutritional deficiencies contribute to mental health degeneration. Strategies for maintaining a nutritionally sound diet are essential in preserving cognitive function and mood stability.

Addiction and Nutrition
Addressing substance abuse involves addressing dietary habits. We explore the bidirectional relationship between addiction and nutrition, offering insights for recovery.

Micronutrients and Mental Health
Micronutrients play a crucial role in cognitive function and emotional stability. Strategies for ensuring adequate intake are discussed alongside evidence from international studies.

International Studies and Findings
Valuable data from international studies inform our understanding of the relationship between diet, nutrition, and mental health.

Nourishing Dietary Modifications
Dietary modifications can support mental health. We explore whole foods and specific nutrients, advocating for a holistic approach to nutrition.

Micronutrient Supplementation
Supplementation may be necessary to address micronutrient deficiencies. Guidance on supplementation under medical supervision is provided.

Mental Health Support
Integrating nutrition with other support modalities ensures a comprehensive approach to mental health.

CHAPTER 51

EMPOWERMENT THROUGH NOURISHMENT

Empowerment is a cornerstone of overall well-being, resonating deeply with individuals striving to lead fulfilling lives. Within this realm, dietary choices emerge as a potent avenue for empowerment, offering a tangible means of shaping one's physical and mental health. This final segment endeavors to illuminate the transformative potential inherent in nutritional support, guiding readers on a journey of comprehension and action. By harnessing the power of informed decision-making and proactive engagement, individuals can cultivate a robust foundation for a healthier, more resilient mind and body.

Introduction to Empowerment through Nourishment:
Empowerment, defined as gaining control and confidence over one's life and circumstances, is profoundly significant in pursuing holistic well-being. Often underestimated in their impact, dietary choices can empower individuals on their wellness journey. This chapter delves into the symbiotic relationship between nourishment and empowerment, elucidating how mindful dietary decisions can catalyze transformative changes in mental and physical health.

The Dual Quest for Understanding and Action: Navigating the intricate mental and nutritional health terrain entails a dual quest for comprehension and implementation. This guide is a beacon of illumination, illuminating the path toward holistic wellness with a blend of compassion and knowledge. By embracing the nuanced interplay of factors shaping mental and nutritional well-being, readers can embark on a voyage towards self-empowerment and recovery, charting a course towards optimal health and vitality.

CRITICAL POINTS FOR CONSIDERATION:

1. **Diet Quality and Mortality among Chinese Adults:**

    - Delve into the findings from the China Health and Nutrition Survey, exploring the association between diet quality and mortality rates among Chinese adults.

    - Highlight critical insights regarding the impact of dietary patterns on long-term health outcomes and mortality risk.

2. **The Mediterranean Diet and Depression:**

    - Examine the findings from the "AMEND" study, which investigated the effects of a Mediterranean diet on depression symptoms in young males.

    - Explore the potential therapeutic benefits of adopting a Mediterranean dietary pattern in mitigating depressive symptoms and enhancing mental well-being.

3. **Comparative Analysis of Dietary Patterns:**

    - Contrast the Mediterranean diet with the Western diet in the context of adolescent depression, drawing insights from current reports and studies.

    - Analyze the divergent effects of these dietary patterns on mental health outcomes, emphasizing the role of dietary quality in shaping psychological well-being.

Expanding Understanding Through Research: By delving into nutritional science and epidemiological research, individuals can deepen their understanding of the intricate connections between diet and well-being. Robust empirical evidence is a guiding beacon, illuminating the path toward informed dietary choices and empowering individuals to take charge of their health destiny.

Practical Applications and Implementation Strategies: With knowledge gleaned from scientific inquiry, readers can translate theoretical insights into tangible action steps. Valuable strategies for integrating nutrient-dense foods, mindful eating

Lorenzi R.Marcos

practices, and dietary diversity into daily life empower individuals to nurture their bodies and minds with intention and purpose.

Holistic Wellness: Fostering a Symphony of Health: Ultimately, the pursuit of empowerment through nourishment transcends the realm of dietary choices, encompassing a holistic approach to wellness. By fostering harmony between mind, body, and spirit, individuals can cultivate a symphony of health that resonates with vitality, resilience, and well-being.

Conclusion: As we journey through the terrain of empowerment through nourishment, let us embrace the transformative potential inherent in our dietary choices. By honoring the symbiotic relationship between nutrition and empowerment, we forge a path toward a brighter, healthier future characterized by vitality, resilience, and the boundless potential of the human spirit.

CHAPTER 52

THE ALLURE OF POWER AND MONEY: A JOURNEY THROUGH NEUROSCIENCE, HISTORY, AND SOCIETY

Power and money have captivated us throughout history, influencing our behavior, choices, and brains. While often perceived as external motivators, the pursuit and possession of these forces set off a chain reaction within us, profoundly shaping our decisions and ultimately reshaping our perceptions of the world. Let's explore the intricate interplay between power, money, and the human experience, drawing upon insights from neuroscience, historical evidence, and the realities of society.

Neurochemical Symphony:
- **Dopamine's Delight:** The acquisition of power and wealth triggers the brain's reward system, releasing dopamine, a neurotransmitter closely associated with pleasure and motivation. This dopamine surge creates a reinforcing loop, intensifying the desire for more power and money, driving individuals to pursue these goals relentlessly.

- **Serotonin's Sway:** Possessing power and wealth can stabilize serotonin levels in the brain, impacting mood regulation and fostering a sense of well-being and self-confidence. This enhanced emotional state further reinforces the allure of pursuing and maintaining positions of power and financial success.

- **Oxytocin's Embrace:** Power and wealth can also influence the release of oxytocin, often called the "bonding hormone." Elevated oxytocin levels foster feelings of trust, social connection, and belonging, thereby solidifying the perceived benefits associated with power and wealth accumulation.

Brain Regions Under the Influence:
- **Prefrontal Cortex:** The dopamine rush associated with power and money can compromise the prefrontal cortex, which is responsible for decision-making and impulse control. This compromised function may lead to risky and

impulsive behavior as individuals prioritize immediate rewards over long-term consequences.

- **Nucleus Accumbens:** The nucleus accumbens, a vital region of the brain's reward circuitry, becomes highly activated in response to acquiring and possessing power and wealth. This heightened activity reinforces the desire for external markers of success, fueling the pursuit of greater power and financial resources.

Amygdala and Power Dynamics:
The amygdala, crucial for processing fear and threat perception, undergoes alterations in individuals with power, potentially resulting in decreased sensitivity. This diminished responsiveness may contribute to heightened aggression and risk-taking behaviors as individuals feel less constrained by perceived threats.

Historical Insights:
- **From Emperors to Entrepreneurs:** Throughout history, individuals in positions of power and wealth have exhibited distinct behaviors and characteristics, shedding light on the psychological impacts of these forces on human behavior.

- **The Rise and Fall of Empires:** Studying the collapse of empires through the lens of power dynamics offers valuable insights into the neurological effects of unrestrained power and the potential pitfalls associated with its pursuit.

- **Philanthropy and Altruism:** Despite the negative connotations often associated with power and money, historical examples of philanthropic endeavors demonstrate their potential for driving positive societal change and improving the lives of others.

Social Observations:
- **Income Inequality and Social Unrest:** Research suggests a correlation between significant income inequality and increased social unrest, underscoring the societal implications of perceived disparities in power and wealth.

- **Status Symbols and Social Climbing:** Societal norms often equate power and money with specific possessions and experiences, fostering a "status chase" that can exacerbate feelings of inadequacy and contribute to addiction and mental health issues.

- **The Power of Education and Empathy:** Educational initiatives that promote critical thinking and empathy play a crucial role in helping individuals navigate the complexities of power and money dynamics, facilitating responsible choices, and fostering positive societal change.

Beyond Judgment:
Understanding the intricate dance between power, money, and our brain chemistry is essential for avoiding simplistic judgments and stereotypes. While acknowledging the undeniable pitfalls associated with their pursuit, recognizing the neurochemical and social influences empowers us to make informed choices and work towards a society where these forces are harnessed for the benefit of all.

Remember:

Pursuing power and money is deeply ingrained in human psychology and social structures. Understanding the neurochemical and social factors empowers us to make informed choices and strive for a more balanced and equitable society.

This exploration provides only a glimpse into the vast and complex world of power and money and their impact on individuals and societies. By examining these themes through the lenses of science, history, and social realities, we can work towards a future where these forces serve as positive catalysts for individual and collective well-being.

CHAPTER 53

UNMASKING THE DANGERS OF NICOTINE ADDICTION

Tobacco use, fueled by nicotine, remains a leading global health concern. Let's delve into its science, shedding light on its dangers and promoting informed choices!

Defining Nicotine Addiction:
- Nicotine addiction, often arising from tobacco use, is characterized by:

  - Compulsive tobacco use: Despite risks and negative consequences, individuals continue to use tobacco products.

  - Loss of control: Difficulty limiting or stopping tobacco use, even when desired.

  - Salient cravings: Intense desires for nicotine that influence behavior.

  - Tolerance: Requiring more nicotine to achieve the same effects.

  - Withdrawal symptoms: Irritability, anxiety, and other physical discomfort when stopping tobacco use.

Neurochemical Impact:
- Nicotine directly impacts key neurotransmitters governing reward, motivation, and learning:

  - Dopamine: Increased dopamine levels trigger pleasure and reinforce repeated tobacco use.

  - Acetylcholine: Stimulates acetylcholine receptors, impacting attention, learning, and mood.

  - Glutamate: Alters glutamate function, contributing to potential changes in cognitive function.

Brain Region Involvement:
- Chronic nicotine exposure affects brain regions crucial for:

    - Prefrontal cortex: Responsible for decision-making, judgment, and impulse control, often compromised in nicotine addiction.

    - Limbic system: This involves emotions, reward processing, and motivation, leading to cravings and emotional dysregulation.

    - Hippocampus: Essential for memory and learning, often negatively impacted by nicotine, causing potential cognitive decline.

Individual Variations:
- While the general neurochemical and brain effects are present, individual responses vary due to:

    - Genetics: Some individuals possess genetic predispositions that increase vulnerability to addiction.

    - Personality: Traits like impulsivity or anxiety can influence susceptibility to nicotine dependence.

    - Environment: Social pressures, accessibility of tobacco products, and cultural norms influence usage patterns.

Long-Term Consequences:
- Chronic nicotine use from tobacco products can lead to severe health problems, including:

    - Cancer: Lung cancer, head and neck cancers, and other types of cancer linked to tobacco use.

    - Heart disease: Increased risk of heart attack, stroke, and other cardiovascular issues.

- Lung disease: COPD, emphysema, and other respiratory problems.
- Other health problems: Weakened immune system, fertility issues, and pregnancy complications.

Social and Behavioral Impact:
- Beyond individual health, nicotine addiction can impact:
    - Relationships: Can strain family ties and social interactions.
    - Financial strain: Costs associated with tobacco products and potential healthcare needs.
    - Social stigma: Societal perceptions can lead to discrimination and judgment.
    - Reduced quality of life: Limited physical activity and potential social isolation.

Beyond Individual Blame:
- Understanding the complex interplay of factors is crucial:
    - Biological factors: Neurochemistry and genetics contribute to vulnerability.
    - Psychological factors: Personality traits and mental health conditions can play a role.
    - Social factors: Marketing, societal norms, and easy access to tobacco products influence usage.

Promote Help-Seeking:
- Nicotine addiction is treatable. Encourage individuals to seek help from:
    - Healthcare professionals: Doctors, therapists, and smoking cessation specialists can offer support and treatment options.

- Support groups: Sharing experiences and connecting with others seeking to quit can be empowering.

- Community resources: Many organizations offer cessation programs and educational materials.

By acknowledging the science and complexities behind nicotine addiction, we can move beyond judgment and create a supportive environment for individuals seeking freedom from tobacco. Remember! This is just one example; you can adapt the framework to explore other addictions, promoting understanding and resources for help.

CHAPTER 53

UNVEILING THE SCIENCE AND SOCIAL IMPACT OF SUGAR ADDICTION

Sugar addiction, often dismissed as mere indulgence, presents a complex issue rooted in biology, psychology, and societal influences. Let's unravel the science behind sugar's grip and its societal impact!

Neurochemical Enticement:
- Dopamine Dance: Sugar triggers a surge in dopamine, the "reward" neurotransmitter, creating a pleasure loop that reinforces continued consumption.

- Serotonin Sway: Sugar can temporarily stabilize serotonin levels, influencing mood and potentially masking underlying emotional issues.

- Glutamate Games: Sugar intake impacts Glutamate, a neurotransmitter associated with learning and memory, creating cravings by associating sugar with positive memories and experiences.

Brain Regions Under Siege:
- Prefrontal Cortex: Responsible for decision-making and impulse control, this region can become compromised by sugar addiction, leading to weakened resistance against cravings.

- Limbic System: This reward and emotion processing hub fuels the cycle of pleasure and cravings associated with sugar intake.

- Hippocampus: Learning and memory functions can be affected by sugar, potentially contributing to the development and perpetuation of addictive behaviors.

Social Factors Fueling the Fire:
- Marketing Blitz: Our environment is bombarded with persuasive marketing that glorifies sugary products, making them seem irresistible and associating them with happiness and fulfillment.

Lorenzi R.Marcos

- Accessibility Overload: Easy access to sugary products everywhere, from supermarkets to workplaces, makes it challenging to avoid temptation, especially for vulnerable individuals.

- Social Pressures: Cultural norms and social gatherings often revolve around sugary treats, creating pressure to partake and potentially fueling addictive behaviors.

Beyond Individual Blame: Sugar addiction is not simply a matter of willpower. Recognizing the complex interplay of biological, psychological, and social factors is crucial for understanding and addressing this issue.

Moving Towards Solutions:
- Promote education and awareness: Raising awareness about the science behind sugar addiction and its societal impact can empower individuals to make informed choices.

- Support healthy alternatives: Encouraging access to nutritious and affordable options can create an environment that fosters more nutritious choices.

- Advocate for regulation: Advocating for rules on the marketing and accessibility of sugary products can help counteract environmental influences contributing to addiction.

Remember: Sugar addiction is a real issue with complex causes. Empathy and understanding are vital in supporting individuals seeking help. Addressing the broader social environment is crucial for long-term solutions. By acknowledging the science and societal factors at play, we can move beyond blame and create a supportive environment that empowers individuals to navigate the complexities of sugar and make informed choices for their well-being.

UNDERSTANDING ALCOHOL ADDICTION:

Alcohol addiction, also known as Alcohol Use Disorder (AUD), is a chronic illness characterized by:

- Compulsive alcohol use: Despite negative consequences, an individual continues to drink excessively.

- Loss of control: Difficulty limiting or resisting alcohol intake.

- Salient cravings: Intense desires for alcohol that influence behavior.

- Tolerance: Requiring more alcohol to achieve the same effects.

- Withdrawal symptoms: Physical and emotional discomfort when stopping alcohol intake.

Neurochemical Impact:

- Alcohol directly impacts critical neurotransmitters that regulate reward, motivation, and learning.

- Dopamine: Increased dopamine levels generate pleasure and reinforce repeated alcohol use.

- GABA: Decreased GABA, an inhibitory neurotransmitter, leads to disinhibition and impaired control.

- Glutamate: Disrupted glutamate function contributes to impaired memory and cognition.

Brain Region Involvement:

- Chronic alcohol use affects various brain regions crucial for decision-making, impulse control, emotions, and memory.

Individual Variations:

- Genetics, personality, and environment play significant roles in individual responses to alcohol addiction.

Long-Term Consequences:

- Prolonged alcohol abuse can lead to severe physical and mental health problems, including liver damage, brain damage, mental health issues, and other health problems.

Social and Behavioral Impact:
- AUD harms relationships, work performance, and finances and leads to risky behaviors.

Promote Help-Seeking:
- AUD is treatable. Encourage individuals to seek help from healthcare professionals, support groups, and community resources.

By acknowledging the science behind alcohol addiction, we can move beyond judgment and foster a supportive environment for individuals seeking recovery.

CHAPTER 54

A GLOBAL SYMPHONY OF SELF: CONDUCTED BY YOU

Reversing the Dialogues of Division:
What if the key to unity lies within our hearts and minds in a world gripped by cultural polarization? I invite you to consider a radical notion – that all meaningful global change begins as an internal revolution, a movement founded on the principles of self-awareness, empathy, and genuine communication! As a Brazilian-Italian holistic coach, I've realized that my most profound transformations occur when I foster a deep understanding of my inner self. It's a silent revolution that echoes a powerful anthem: self-knowledge not only liberates the individual, but it also has the potential to heal the divisions of society.

The Somatic Symphony: Understanding Your Body's Language:
Let's embark on a journey of profound exploration, where the body is our first instrument. How often do we stop to listen to the intricate melodies that our bodies compose? From the rise and fall of the breath to the pulse of our heartbeat, these rhythms paint a picture of our inner state. As a certified personal trainer, I've witnessed the transformative power of bodily awareness. It is the root chakra of our being, the foundation upon which self-mastery is built. I'll guide you through techniques that tune your body to the frequency of health and vitality, preparing you to interlace your physical self with the more extraordinary global tapestry.

Harmonizing the Mind: Stoicism and Hermeticism in the Modern Age:
The mind, our most potent conductor, requires mastery no less than the body. The ancient philosophies of stoicism and hermeticism provide the baton to orchestrate our thoughts and perceptions. By inviting their timeless wisdom into our lives, we learn to craft a narrative uncontested by the storms of modern life. I'll share excerpts from my journey when these philosophies

illuminate paths where none existed before and guide you through practices that fortify the mind and sharpen its focus.

Instruments of Virtue: Playing the Notes of Integrity:
At the symphony's heart lies the concept of virtue – the moral markers that guide our actions. In a world that often celebrates expediency over integrity, how can we ensure our conduct is a testimony to our highest self? We will explore the cardinal virtues of wisdom, courage, justice, and temperance, aligning them as the compass that points us toward personal fulfillment and as contributors to the greater good.

An Overture of Knowledge: Seeking the Truth of Our Existence:

Knowledge is the culmination of the self's pursuit, the point where understanding becomes actionable insight. In absorbing knowledge, we accept the responsibility to reflect that truth daily. We will delve into the vast human experience and research library, uniting intellectual and practical pursuits to shape a more empowered existence.

The Dialogue of Peace: Channeling Conflict into Connection:
Conflict is inevitable, yet our perspective can transform it from a fork in the road to a knot in the fabric of society. Through mindful communication and a willingness to listen, we can dissolve barriers and understand that we bear the same human essence beneath our diversity. In this unity, we find peace, and in this peace, we establish the conditions for global harmony.

Epilogue: Orchestrating Change from Within:
The global symphony I propose is not a solo endeavor; it requires everyone to take up the baton and play their part. Through self-understanding, we can each become a conductor, leading movements that resonate with universal truths. With every note, we contribute to a movement that transcends borders, languages, and cultures—a testament to the power of the internal revolution and its profound implications for a world replete with harmony and understanding.

In the noisy orchestra of life, find your silence! It is there, in the stillness, that we truly begin to play.

CHAPTER 55

WE ARE WHAT WE EAT AND BECOME WHAT WE HEAR AND SEE

In an age where digital consumption is as regular as our daily meals, we must recognize what we put into our bodies and what we feed our brains. Our audio-visual content can significantly affect our cognitive functions and potentially lead to unconscious behaviors. This blog post unravels the influence of sounds, songs, and visual communication on brain function and underscores the importance of mindful digital content consumption, especially among today's youth.

The Power of Sound and Music

Have you ever noticed how a particular song can alter your mood, energize you, or even soothe your nerves? There's science behind this phenomenon. Sounds and music can activate the brain's reward systems, releasing neurotransmitters like dopamine that make us feel good. Moreover, repetitive exposure to certain types of music can form associations in our brains, often leading to behavioral changes without our conscious awareness.

In advertising and marketing, experts have long utilized these understandings to influence consumer behavior. Fast-paced, upbeat music in stores can encourage quick decision-making, while a slower tempo might be used in a spa setting to promote relaxation.

Visual Stimuli and Brain Function

Visual content, particularly short-form videos popularized on social media platforms, is designed to capture attention instantaneously. The rapid shift in scenes and information in these videos can condition the brain to expect a constant stream of stimulation, diminishing attention spans and altering how data is processed and retained. Furthermore, repetitive visual and digital content themes can shape our perceptions and beliefs.

The tactic is known as priming. Once primed, viewers may unconsciously adopt certain behaviors or attitudes mirrored in their consumed content.

The Importance of Content Choice

With youth's developing brains being remarkably malleable, the choice of digital content becomes paramount. Young viewers are more susceptible to the suggestive power of the audio-visual material they're exposed to daily. Their entertainment can reinforce specific neural pathways, influencing everything from language acquisition to social behaviors. The crux lies in increasing awareness that we might inadvertently allow it to shape who we become when we absorb content mindlessly. Therefore, it's important for consumers—and parents of young consumers—to be intentional about their content choices.

SOCIAL MEDIA: A DOUBLE-EDGED SWORD

While social media can be a tremendous source of learning, inspiration, and connectivity, it can just as quickly be an echo chamber for negative influencers. The ubiquity of social platforms bestows upon them a significant responsibility to moderate and curate content conducive to positive reinforcement and genuine information sharing.

Key Takeaways for Digital Content Consumers

- Be Conscious of What You Consume: Treat digital content consumption with the same discernment as dietary choices!

- Practice Moderation: Balance is essential. Overexposure to a specific type of content can have inadvertent behavioral ramifications.

- Seek Diverse Perspectives: Diversification can prevent the formation of echo chambers and promote critical thinking.

- Encourage Healthy Habits in Youth: Educate younger viewers on the importance of selective content consumption and the potential impact of their digital diets!

Conclusion

In a world inundated with digital content, our role as consumers is more active than passive. It's essential to approach the media we digest with a critical eye, understanding that our brains are listening, watching, and, quite literally, being shaped by what we hear and see. As we continually navigate the sea of digital content, let's strive for choices that nurture rather than numb our cognitive faculties, enlighten instead of manipulate, and celebrate the autonomy of our thought processes! Remember! The path to cognitive autonomy and healthier social media habits begins with a simple yet potent practice: choice. (TOOLBOX N23080639MRLT)

CHAPTER 56

SIMPLE DIY ART PROJECTS FOR STRESS RELIEF AND FOCUS DEVELOPMENT

Beyond the creative fun, simple DIY art projects offer surprising benefits for your brain, community, and well-being. Engaging in these activities:

1. **Boosts Neuroplasticity:** Coloring and origami stimulate new neural connections, enhancing focus, memory, and cognitive flexibility.

2. **Fosters Community Connection:** Sharing your creations online or participating in local art workshops fosters connection and a sense of belonging.

3. **Promotes Mindfulness:** Focusing on the present moment while doodling or sculpting can reduce stress and improve overall well-being.

Dive into the world of DIY art and unlock a treasure trove of benefits for your mind, body, and community!

- **Coloring:** This classic activity is effective for both adults and children. Choose coloring books with intricate patterns, mandalas for added focus, or even color-printed images from magazines or online!

- **Doodling:** Grab a pen, pencil, or marker and let your hand wander freely on paper! This helps quiet the mind and promote relaxation. You can also try structured doodles like Zentangles or patterns.

- **Nature Mandala Creation:** Gather natural materials like leaves, flowers, pebbles, and twigs and arrange them flat to create a visually pleasing and calming mandala. This activity connects you with nature while fostering creativity and focus.

- **Origami:** Folding paper into intricate shapes requires concentration and precision, making it a great way to train your focus while creating beautiful figures.

- **Play-Doh Sculpting:** Squishing, molding, and shaping Play-Doh is a tactile experience that can be incredibly calming and relieving. Allow yourself to be creative and playful!

- **Sand Art:** Create mesmerizing sand art in a bottle or tray! Layer different-colored sand and use tools or fingers to swirl and create patterns. This activity is visually captivating and provides a sense of accomplishment.

- **Mindful Drawing:** Set a timer for 5-10 minutes and focus on drawing a specific object from life, like a flower or a cup! Pay close attention to details and textures, allowing yourself to be fully present in the moment!

- **Gratitude Jar:** Decorate a jar and fill it with slips of paper where you write down things you are grateful for! Write whenever you feel overwhelmed or stressed, and take a moment to read through these reminders of positivity!

- **Mandala Rock Painting:** Collect smooth rocks and paint them with intricate designs, patterns, or mandalas! This activity combines the benefits of mindfulness with the joy of creating something beautiful.

- **Nature Photography:** Go for a nature walk and capture the beauty of the surroundings through your camera (phone or dedicated camera)! Focus on specific details like textures, patterns, or exciting angles! This practice promotes mindfulness and appreciation for nature.

A 2018 Frontiers in Human Neuroscience study found that regular coloring increases brain activity in memory, attention, and visual processing regions. <u>Source</u> This suggests the potential for improved cognitive function.

A 2018 "Frontiers in Psychology" study found that mindful art activities can promote present-moment awareness and emotional regulation, leading to increased well-being. Source

Conclusion

In conclusion, navigating the complexities of modern life can be daunting. Just as a lion in the savanna wouldn't unquestioningly accept any food source or attempt a hunt without honing its skills, humans must actively understand and prioritize our health. This journey begins with awareness. How often do we truly consider the impact of our choices on our physical and mental well-being?

Imagine a lion cub who relies solely on instinct, ignoring the wisdom of its experienced pride. It might attempt a risky jump before its muscles are developed or consume a seemingly attractive plant, unaware of its toxicity. Similarly, investing in our health knowledge can have beneficial consequences.

Consider prioritizing your health as acquiring the necessary skills for a successful life! Just as a lion wouldn't expect to hunt without training its body, we can't expect to navigate life's challenges without a foundation of knowledge and self-care practices. This learning process ideally begins in our youth, nurtured by guidance from parents and educators. By fostering a culture of health awareness from a young age, we empower individuals to make informed choices about their well-being.

BIOGRAPHY OF HISTORICAL AND PRESENT MOST RELEVANT MASTERS OF ALL TIMES

Leonardo da Vinci (1452-1519):
The quintessential Renaissance Man, da Vinci excelled as a painter, sculptor, inventor, engineer, scientist, and anatomist. His iconic works like the Mona Lisa and The Last Supper inspire awe, while his notebooks reveal a mind far ahead of its time, filled with groundbreaking ideas in mechanics, optics, and anatomy.

Nikola Tesla (1856-1943):
A prolific inventor and electrical engineer, Tesla's innovations revolutionized modern life. He is best known for developing alternating current (AC) electricity, the foundation of our modern power grids, and for his pioneering work in wireless communication and robotics. Tesla's visionary ideas continue to influence technology today.

Harriet Tubman (c. 1822 – 1913):
A courageous conductor on the Underground Railroad, Tubman risked her life to guide enslaved people to freedom before the Civil War. Nicknamed "Moses," she led 13 missions and freed over 70 enslaved people. Tubman's bravery and unwavering fight for freedom continue to inspire generations as a symbol of resilience and resistance.

Lúcia Helena Galvão (1963-present):
A contemporary Brazilian philosopher, Lúcia Helena Galvão is a professor and a leading figure in the organization New Acropolis. Her work applies philosophical ideas to everyday life, drawing on various traditions, including Stoicism, Hermeticism, and Eastern philosophies. She offers courses and lectures on happiness, ethics, and finding meaning in life. While not as widely known as the other figures on this list, her work is influential in Brazil and beyond.

Marcus Aurelius (121-180 AD):
Roman emperor and Stoic philosopher Marcus Aurelius is renowned for his "Meditations," a collection of personal writings offering guidance on living a virtuous life. Stoicism emphasizes reason, duty, and accepting what is outside our control. Marcus Aurelius' reflections on mortality, self-discipline, and finding purpose continue to resonate with readers today.

Seneca (4 BC-65 AD):
A prominent Roman statesman, playwright, and Stoic philosopher, Seneca explored themes of virtue, happiness, and the pursuit of a meaningful life. His writings emphasize the importance of reason, self-control, and overcoming negative emotions. Seneca's letters offer practical advice for living a good life despite challenges.

Epictetus (50-130 AD):
A Greek Stoic philosopher, Epictetus believed that true happiness comes from focusing on what we can control—our thoughts and actions—rather than external circumstances. His teachings emphasize personal responsibility, accepting what is beyond our control, and living virtuously. Although Epictetus wrote no books, his student Arrian compiled his discourses and remained influential.

Socrates (470-399 BC):
A pivotal figure in the history of Western philosophy, Socrates is known for his method of inquiry, the Socratic Method, which uses questioning to stimulate critical thinking and expose faulty reasoning. He believed actual knowledge comes from self-examination and emphasized the importance of living a virtuous life. While Socrates wrote nothing himself, his ideas were preserved through the writings of his students, particularly Plato.

Plato (428/427-348/347 BC):
A student of Socrates, Plato is considered one of the most influential philosophers in history. He founded the Academy, the first institution of higher learning in the Western world. Plato's dialogues explore various topics, including ethics, politics, metaphysics, and epistemology. His theory of Forms, which posits a realm of perfect ideal Forms that our world imperfectly reflects, remains a cornerstone of Western philosophical thought.

Mohandas Gandhi (1869-1948):
Mahatma Gandhi, meaning "Great Soul," was the preeminent leader of Indian nationalism in British-ruled India. Employing nonviolent civil disobedience, Gandhi led India to independence and inspired movements for civil rights and freedom worldwide. His philosophy of Satyagraha, meaning "truth force," emphasized truth, nonviolence, and love as the means to achieve social change.

Jesus of Nazareth (c. 4 BC – c. 30 AD):
The central figure of Christianity, Christians revered Jesus as the Son of God. His teachings on love, forgiveness, and compassion continue influencing billions worldwide. The Gospels, the foundational texts of Christianity, detail Jesus' life, ministry, miracles, and teachings, emphasizing themes of salvation, redemption, and eternal life.

Siddhartha Gautama (c. 563 BCE – c. 483 BCE):
The founder of Buddhism, Siddhartha Gautama, also known as the Buddha, meaning "Awakened One," experienced a spiritual awakening after a lifetime of seeking to understand suffering. His teachings focus on the Four Noble Truths, a path to end suffering through enlightenment. Buddhism emphasizes mindfulness, meditation, and moral living to attain liberation from suffering.

ABOUT THE AUTHOR

Originating from the tranquil landscapes of a Brazilian hamlet, Lorenzi R. Marcos found solace amidst the masterpieces of Renaissance art and the rich narratives echoing through its cobblestone. This early immersion birthed a genuine ardor for history, biology, and the enigmatic depths of human existence.

At a mere 14 years old, Lorenzi's life took an unexpected turn, thrusting them into the bustling heart of Brasilia, where independence became their reluctant companion. This pivotal juncture catalyzed a journey that saw them traverse continents, with Italy beckoning at 18 as the first stop on a nomadic odyssey spanning six distinct countries over 24 dynamic years.

Amidst the kaleidoscope of cultural encounters, Lorenzi found themselves grappling with an ever-present sense of solitude, igniting an insatiable hunger for understanding human complexities. Thus began a quest that unfolded over a decade, delving deep into philosophy, neuroscience, and the emotive expressions of art, each offering a unique prism to explore the labyrinth of self.

The road to self-awareness was fraught with obstacles, from the treacherous pitfalls of misinformation to the suffocating embrace of societal expectations. Yet, with unwavering resolve, Lorenzi confronted these challenges head-on, peeling away layers of illusion and delusion to uncover the radiant truth within.

Through the crucible of self-discovery, Lorenzi emerged, shedding the shackles of addiction, disillusionment, and negativity. In their wake, they left a legacy of reverence for all life forms and an unyielding commitment to global enlightenment and universal equity. Thus, their transformative journey became a personal triumph and a beacon of hope for all seeking liberation from the shadows of ignorance and prejudice.

APPRECIATION AND ACCREDITATION
To Pakistan Umar Arif and Valmira Cristina de Andrade:

The essence of this book owes much to the remarkable contributions of Pakistan Umar Arif and Valmira Cristina de Andrade. Their wealth of experience and visionary perspectives have laid a robust groundwork for the ideas presented in these pages, shaping the very fabric of our narrative.

A special acknowledgment extends to my translator, whose adept handling of language nuances has seamlessly bridged cultures, ensuring an inclusive reading experience for diverse audiences.

Heartfelt appreciation goes out to the talented individuals behind the scenes — the editor, the graphic designer, and the Publisher — who have poured their expertise and passion into bringing this book to fruition. Their meticulous attention to detail and creative flair have transformed my manuscript into a captivating work of art, a testament to collaborative excellence.

MY GRATITUDE TO DR. VALMIRA CRISTINA DE ANDRADE AND MR. UMAR (THE CONTRIBUTORS)

To Dr. Valmira Cristina de Andrade and Mr. Umar:

With deep appreciation, I extend my heartfelt gratitude to Dr. Valmira Cristina de Andrade and Mr. Umar for their invaluable contributions to my forthcoming book. Dr. Andrade, a luminary in nutrition, sports neuroscience, and behavior change, has illuminated our project with her visionary approach encapsulated in "Emagrecidamente." Her dedication to sustainable weight management strategies inspires readers worldwide to embrace holistic well-being.

Similarly, Mr. Umar, a distinguished ISSA personal trainer and nutrition coach, has enriched our endeavor with his expertise tailored to the unique needs of men aged 30 to 40. His commitment to empowering individuals with the tools for optimal health underscores the transformative potential of personalized fitness and nutrition guidance.

Their unwavering dedication and genuine concern for others exemplify the spirit of collaboration essential for effecting positive change in global fitness and nutrition practices. Their voices lend credence to our shared vision of a healthier world where science and empathy converge to nurture holistic wellness.

Reach out to them on this social handle: LinkedIn: http://linkedin.com/in/umar-arif-a534b13b (Mr. Umar)

INSTAGRAM HANDLE @umarthecoach (Mr. Umar)

Mail address: umarthefitnesscoach@gmail.com (Mr. Umar)

INSTAGRAM HANDLE @nutricionista.val.andrade (Dr. Valmira Cristina de Andrade)

c nutricionistavalmiraandrade@gmail.com

With sincere appreciation,

Lorenzi R. Marcos.

MY GRATITUDE TO NIGEL AND BEATRIZ JARVIS (TRANSLATOR)

To Nigel and Beatriz Jarvis:

Nigel and Beatriz Jarvis stand as unparalleled artisans in the vibrant tapestry of literary creation, weaving language into a symphony of meaning. Their dedication to the craft of translation transformed my book from mere words on a page into a living, breathing entity that resonates with readers across cultures.

Nigel and Beatriz's expertise in online English teaching, translations, and meticulous proofreading is remarkable. Their passion for history and education, exemplified by Nigel's establishment of the Jarvis Mixed Martial Arts, is a testament to their commitment to excellence in all endeavors. Linked with the renowned Magda Institute in Reseda, California, they have honed their skills to perfection, ensuring that every word and nuance is captured with precision and grace.

Beyond their professional accomplishments, Nigel and Beatriz's hearts beat with compassion for animal welfare. Their unwavering dedication to the well-being of rescued pets reflects a kindness that extends far beyond the pages of any book.

As I embark on this new chapter in Canada, I am profoundly grateful for Nigel and Beatriz's invaluable contributions to my work. Their talent, diligence, and unwavering support have breathed life into my words, allowing them to soar across borders and touch readers' hearts worldwide.

Reach out on mail : jarvisalves.uk@gmail.com

With sincere appreciation,

Lorenzi R. Marcos.

MY GRATITUDE KEHINDE AKINOLA (PUBLISHER)

Dear Kehinde Akinola:

I am writing to express my most profound appreciation and gratitude for the incredible journey we've embarked upon together. Your unwavering support, dedication, and belief in my book have transformed it from mere words on paper to a vibrant, living entity.

From the first moment we connected, your passion for literature and commitment to nurturing authors' voices shone through. Your meticulous attention to detail and invaluable insights have elevated my work beyond what I imagined possible.

I am profoundly grateful for your trust in me and the countless hours you and your team devoted to bringing my vision to life. Your expertise in the publishing industry, coupled with your unwavering encouragement, has been the driving force behind the success of my book.

Thank you for championing my story and believing in its power to resonate with readers. Your contributions have shaped my book and enriched the lives of those who have had the privilege of experiencing it.

I am immensely proud to be associated with such a reputable and esteemed publisher, and I look forward to continuing our collaboration in future endeavors.

Reach out on mail : classiknn@gmail.com

Facebook: Akinola Ella (Caroline)

With most profound appreciation and admiration,

Lorenzi R. Marcos.

I am deeply grateful for their support and the invaluable perspectives they have shared.

CREDENTIALS AND EXPERTISE

Lorenzi R. Marcos holds a prestigious certification from the American Council on Exercise as a Personal Trainer specializing in fitness, postural corrections, behavior modification, and weight management. Additionally, He excels as a mindfulness coach and a culinary artist specializing in plant-based cuisine, deriving immense joy from crafting delectable vegetarian dishes.

Inspired by a diverse array of mentors, including Leonardo da Vinci, Nikola Tesla, Harriet Tubman, Mahatma Gandhi, Marcus Aurelius, Socrates, Seneca, Jesus, and Buddha, Lorenzi R. Marcos has explored over 20 distinct professions and embarked on exploratory journeys to over 50 countries across four continents. This rich tapestry of experiences has instilled a profound appreciation for multiculturalism and an unwavering love for all living beings.

THE BOOK'S PURPOSE

This book serves as a call to action, urging readers to comprehend their bodies, nurture them with proper fuel, and adopt habits conducive to optimal health. Just as a skilled lion reigns supreme in the savanna, individuals with knowledge and healthy practices become formidable forces in shaping their destinies. Through self-discovery and prioritizing well-being, this book aims to be a guiding light toward a vibrant and fulfilling life.

THE OBJECTIVE OF THE BOOK

Lorenzi R. Marcos's overarching objective in this literary endeavor is to empower individuals to break free from the constraints of addiction and misinformation. He aspires to guide readers on their transformative journeys of self-discovery and positive change by providing them with essential tools and unwavering support. This endeavor transcends victimhood narratives, advocating instead for the reclamation of personal agency and the transformative potential of knowledge and self-awareness.

BILL OF RIGHT KNOW THYSELF

BLACK WHITE & SHADOWS OF HUMANITY
HEALTH HERITAGE

NEUROSCIENCE
PHILOSOPHY
HUMANITY

CONGRATULATIONS TO YOU
AS YOU DISCOVER

THE BILL OF RIGHTS. KNOW
THYSELF

SPECIAL GREETING FROM Lorenzi R. Marcos

www.ingramcontent.com/pod-product-compliance
Lightning Source LLC
Chambersburg PA
CBHW081147270326
41930CB00014B/3063